W9-AVS-348

EXPECTING
TROUBLE

EXPECTING TROUBLE

▼

The Myth of Prenatal Care in America

THOMAS H. STRONG, JR., M.D.

NEW YORK UNIVERSITY PRESS
New York and London

NEW YORK UNIVERSITY PRESS
New York and London

© 2000 by New York University
All rights reserved.

Library of Congress Cataloging-in-Publication Data
Strong, Thomas H.
Expecting trouble : the myth of prenatal care in America / Thomas H.
Strong, Jr.
p.   cm.
Includes bibliographical references (p.   ) and index.
ISBN 0-8147-9767-9 (cloth : acid-free paper)
1. Prenatal care—United States.   I. Title.
RG960 .S77 2000
362.1'9824'0973—dc21   00-008927

New York University Press books are printed on acid-free paper,
and their binding materials are chosen for strength and durability.

Manufactured in the United States of America
10 9 8 7 6 5 4 3 2 1

This book is dedicated to my father,
Dr. Thomas H. Strong (1925–1997),
the bravest man I've ever known.
Tempus fugit, Dad.

Contents

Acknowledgments

Since I cannot type, I am very grateful to Lois J. McConville, Julie M. Hector, Susan S. Weisman, and Patricia L. Polich for transcribing my handwritten notes.

This book is entirely my own. My partners at Phoenix Perinatal Associates do not necessarily agree with or endorse its premise or thesis.

1. Heresy: Sowing the Seeds of Change

Little is done during conventional prenatal care that could be expected to influence birthweight or gestational age at birth in any direct fashion.[1]
—Phillip G. Stubblefield, University of Vermont

The Emperor Has No Clothes

One evening at Good Samaritan Regional Medical Center in Phoenix, I deliver a baby who is fifteen weeks premature. A loaf of raisin bread weighs more than he does. The boy struggles for air with heaving chest movements that resemble slow-motion hiccups and his skin is so thin and waxy that he's rendered translucent. Weeks later when the child is discharged from the hospital, he's blind, experiences recurring seizures, and has all the signs of profound mental retardation. Shortly after his first birthday, his mother prematurely delivers his brother.

I can't reconcile why things like this happen, but in America, they happen too often. After all, when an expectant mother seeks prenatal care, shouldn't she and her child benefit from the effort? Isn't it inevitable that those who fail to secure prenatal care will fare less well than their medically supervised counterparts? If you think so, I've got a message for you: the woman mentioned above had early, ample prenatal care.

Let me introduce myself. I am a third generation doctor and a second generation obstetrician. My entire professional career has centered around prenatal care. All of my days—and many of my nights—have been spent caring for expectant mothers. I'm a Clinical Assistant Professor in Obstetrics and Gynecology at universities in two states, a reviewer for five different medical journals and a published researcher, and the singular lesson I've learned from my experience is that most American women are unduly anxious about their chances of developing pregnancy complications and simultaneously overoptimistic about our ability to cure them. Yet to most families and policymakers, the connection between maternity care and a

1

beautiful birthing experience is patently obvious; a forgone conclusion despite the fact that many of the benefits ascribed to prenatal care are unsupported by medical research.

2

Who Should Read This Book and Why

Prenatal care is second only to the general medical examination as the most accessed "preventive" healthcare service in the United States.[2] Thus, *Expecting Trouble* was written to cast light on the looming blind spot which exists in our collective view of American prenatal care. It is intended primarily for parents and healthcare policymakers; in other words, for those who partake of prenatal care and for those most capable of changing it. With maternity statistics that approach those of some underdeveloped nations, it's time to scrutinize the system to which we entrust pregnant women. Expectant parents can no longer afford uncritical acceptance of American-style prenatal care. For them, this is required reading, and it's going to be upsetting. For policymakers, *Expecting Trouble* will be a rude awakening, calling into question many of the prevailing assumptions which have driven our country's maternity healthcare for decades. Indeed, a secondary aim of *Expecting Trouble* is to dispel the many popular misconceptions about prenatal care by providing a realistic, scientifically supported account of what it can, and more importantly, what it cannot do for our mothers. To be clear, this is not a book against prenatal care, and it does not argue that prenatal care cannot be beneficial. But our current system does not serve our children or our mothers as well as it could. This book aims to show what prenatal care simply cannot do, and how it can better focus its energies in order to be as beneficial as possible. Specifically, this book will address:

- The most glaring deficiencies and inconsistencies of American prenatal care.
- The need for more realistic expectations about prenatal care.
- Specific questions that mothers/parents should be asking.
- The larger policy issues regarding prenatal care and women's health.

You are here against terrible odds: the probability that any of your mother's seven million eggs would fuse with any one of the your father's 50 billion sperm to create the entity known as "you" was roughly 1 in 350,000,000,000,000,000. If that much money was placed in a pile, every person on earth could take seven million dollars from it. And as if the chances for your existence weren't already minuscule, the same odds applied to each of your forebearers. Whether by provenance or incredible luck, your very being is miraculous. Human reproduction is both simple and complex, life-giving and life-threatening. It ensures that only one fetus at a time is conceived 99 percent of the time. It ensures that 97 percent of all fetuses will be free of major structural or genetic abnormalities. Moreover, when it's time to be born, our reproductive system makes sure that 97 percent of us deliver head first and that our umbilical cords are short enough to keep us from striking the ground when we bungee dive from our mothers' climate-controlled wombs. It's a finely tuned system. In most cases, the outcome of a given pregnancy—however good or bad—is unrelated to the care provided by doctors. Frequently, they're hapless bystanders; heroes if all goes well or malpractice defendants if it doesn't. A system so inherently efficient and successful is a boon to the care provider, culminating well sufficiently often to provide the illusion that he/she has favorably impacted the outcome. But it's this same highly evolved system that usually renders the services of obstetricians or midwives unnecessary.

The notion that a natural, ages-old process needs our "guidance" reflects an attitude less well evolved than the process we are claiming to help; the perceived need for ritualized medical care during pregnancy is more cultural than medical. According to a noted anthropologist, the single most powerful influence on a society's maternity system is its concept of pregnancy and birth.[3] And in America, pregnancy is considered a disability despite the fact that it is a self-limited, non-communicable, and frequently gratifying condition unlike any other for which medical specialists exist. Sadly, however, pregnancy has become a predicament from which the "patient" must be delivered—a notion fostered daily with assertions that prenatal care somehow fortifies gestation.

America's obstetric history is a manifestation of many entrenched economic and social problems. The politically expedient proposition that prenatal care can provide a simple remedy to potential problems at birth isn't supported by the available evidence and reveals just how poorly we understand the present state of affairs. But in America, flimsy scientific support for prenatal care has been swamped by advocates' calls for its expansion. As happens with too many noble causes, the original intent of prenatal care has been subordinated to the system it engendered. American mothers are now secondary to the promotion of political careers, academic ascension, and outright greed.

Prenatal Care: What Is It?

4   **While we unhesitatingly accept the often reiterated aim of [prenatal] care as a means of reducing . . . mortality, what exactly [prenatal] care consists of and how it works has been less clear to us."[4]**
                      —British Social Services, Committee Report

Picture yourself as a young woman in good health who's pregnant for the first time. If your prenatal care were similar to that received by many expectant American mothers, each clinic visit would entail a quick assessment of your vital signs, urine, uterus, and fetal heartbeat, a regimen that's remained essentially unchanged since very early this century when hypertensive problems like preeclampsia were the most dreaded of pregnancy complications. Occasionally, you'd undergo a pelvic or ultrasound examination. But the lion's share of each well-oiled appointment would be conducted by a nurse, technician, or other non-physician (not that this is a problem—as we'll see later, taking doctors out of the loop for low-risk pregnancies may have its merits). Sometimes your visit would culminate with a brief appearance by your venerable but hasty obstetrician, but your interaction with him or her would occupy less time than it takes to play a short hole of golf. What place do these regimens have in contemporary obstetrics? Let's look at the components of the typical prenatal visit individually:

Maternal Vital Signs. Virtually every encounter with any healthcare provider entails an assessment of one's vital signs. When it comes to prenatal care, we focus on maternal weight and blood pressure because when a complication such as preeclampsia develops, both weight and blood pressure are often abnormally elevated. Indeed, the assessment of a mother's vital signs is a cheap, useful tool. But as will be discussed later, this technique doesn't prevent preeclampsia, though it allows us to detect the problem. Of all the components of a prenatal care visit, however, assessment of maternal vital signs is one of the bigger "bangs for the buck."

Urinalysis. At each prenatal visit, a mother's urine is routinely evaluated for the presence of protein, yet another sign of preeclampsia. But does this long-lived practice make a difference? A study by Dr. Robert K. Gribble at the Marshfield Clinic in Marshfield, Wisconsin, would suggest not.[5] After studying over 3,200 pregnant women, Dr. Gribble found that among low-risk patients with no clear evidence of hypertensive problems, routine urine screening at each prenatal visit did not provide any clinically important information. Moreover, at least three other studies failed to find any value for such screening in low-risk mothers.[6-8]

Uterine Measurement. As the fetus grows, so grows the uterus. Thus, one should be able to indirectly evaluate fetal growth by monitoring the growth of the uterus. But in actuality, it's a fairly unreliable technique—so much so that Dr. J. Sikorski found that when hospitals in London, England, implemented an experimental trial of reduced prenatal visits (i.e., fewer opportunities to measure the uterus), there was a reduction in the rate of false diagnoses of growth-stunted fetuses.[9] Monitoring the growth of the uterus is an inexpensive, simple, and noninvasive tool, and it probably does find the occasional undergrown or overgrown baby. But due to its imprecision, its relative contribution to the overall well-being of mothers and fetuses is small. Worse, it may lead to unnecessary interventions.

Fetal Heart Rate. Listening for the fetal heartbeat accomplishes one goal: it determines if the fetus is alive or not. Period. Listening to the fetal heartbeat rarely detects fetal distress and doesn't improve fetal outcomes.

Customary Laboratory Tests. A number of laboratory tests are administered at various times during pregnancy. At the first prenatal visit, an initial battery of tests is performed to look for evidence of anemia, hepatitis B, syphilis, and isoimmunization, and to determine the mother's blood type. HIV screening is also offered at many prenatal clinics. During this visit, the pregnant woman typically also receives a Pap smear and screens for gonorrhea, chlamydia, and urinary tract infections. Later in gestation, the mother will be offered a test (maternal serum alpha-fetoprotein analysis) which screens for certain types of fetal anomalies, and finally, a screen for gestational diabetes will be administered. Because these tests are minimally invasive, they pose little risk to the mother and do, on occasion, identify problems which merit further attention.

Throughout most of its history, obstetrics hasn't been a terribly scientific discipline. Earlier this century, prenatal regimens did not proceed from sound medical research but instead were issued by the decree of influential obstetric leaders. It was of little consequence to the obstetric ascendancy of the day that much of what they promulgated was at best, worthless and at worst, disfiguring or dangerous. To deal with hypertensive complications in the previous century, for example, pregnant women were sometimes advised to have their breasts amputated.[10] For morning sickness earlier this century, cocaine was the treatment of choice in some quarters. Unfortunately, few mothers or healthcare providers are sufficiently well-informed to counter the authoritative-sounding claims of modern obstetrics. The perception that contemporary American prenatal care is an essential, unequivocally valuable commodity for our mothers persists because too few of us are capable of discerning good intentions from genuine medical knowledge.

Almost one hundred years after its advent, it's still a mystery as to what actually constitutes prenatal care, nor do we know which aspects of prenatal care really confer benefit to our mothers. Even the Institute of Medicine itself acknowledges that the term "prenatal care" represents an inexact collection of interactions and procedures which focuses more upon the total number of prenatal care visits than on the actual content or quality of those visits.[11] To exemplify how pervasive the confusion is, Dr. Michael J. Hughey at Northwestern University conducted a detailed survey regarding the specific content of prenatal care.[12] Upon completion of his study of twenty-six medical groups in Minneapolis-St. Paul, Dr. Hughey found that even within this fairly small geographic area, there was considerable disagreement regarding the elements of even the most basic type of prenatal care. On a larger scale, a fair amount of inconsistency exists between the U.S. Preventive Services Task Force and the Public Service Expert Panel on the Content of Prenatal Care regarding their recommendations about the nature and delivery of prenatal healthcare services in the United States.[13] Significant differences exist between the two sets of guidelines regarding the organization of care, clinical testing and screening, and pregnancy education.

Quantity vs. Quality

After reviewing data from the 1980 National Natality Survey, Dr. Milton Kotelchuck of the University of North Carolina cautioned against proposals to reduce U.S. infant mortality which merely recommend more prenatal visits: "The efficacy of prenatal care interventions rather than access may be the important issue for these women."[14] Yet to this day, most American women visit their obstetricians an average of fourteen times during their pregnancies, a frequency first established decades ago. Critics of American prenatal care have long deprecated the many inconvenient and unproductive visits that healthy, symptomless mothers make to their doctors. Nevertheless, the American College of Obstetricians and Gynecologists and the American Academy of Pediatrics still recommend thirteen to fourteen prenatal visits for each pregnant woman.[15] By comparison, the average number of prenatal care visits in Europe is generally less than in the United States, though each of the countries listed below has a *lower* infant mortality rate than that of the United States:[16]

7

	Average Number of Visits
Denmark	8
Finland	14
France	6
(West) Germany	9
Luxembourg	5
Netherlands	13
Sweden	14
Switzerland	5

Reprinted by permission of Blackwell Science, Inc., from B. Blondel, "Some Characteristics of Antenatal Care in 13 European Countries." *British Journal of Obstetrics and Gynecology* 92(1985)565.

Based on the experience of Western Europe, it appears that quantity of care is not a reliable reflection of overall quality. Yet it's quantity that occupies a central theme in the catechism of American maternity care, even though the majority of low-birthweight babies in this country are born to women with adequate or better prenatal care, quantitatively speaking.[17] A nineteen-year review of pregnancy outcomes in England and France revealed no differences between these countries despite the fact that English mothers made twice as many prenatal visits as their French counterparts.[18] Even the National Institute of Health advises that the number of prenatal visits for low-risk mothers should be reduced to eight or ten—and that healthy mothers should have even fewer.[19] Over ten years ago, a published review of prenatal care concluded that the scope and content of prenatal care are more important than the quantity of care. More recently, Dr. Mark A. Binstock of the University of California in Los Angeles found that low-risk mothers who make fewer prenatal visits had equally good outcomes as those receiving traditional care.[20] But perhaps the best study

8

on this subject was conducted by Dr. Paul Buescher at the North Carolina State Center for Health Statistics who made the surprising discovery that mothers who received prenatal care from nurses at a public health clinic had significantly fewer low-birthweight babies than did those who received prenatal care from private physicians.[21] Dr. Buescher's observations are even more remarkable given that mothers receiving care from the public health clinics also made fewer prenatal visits than those receiving care from private doctors. Yet, undaunted, we continue to promulgate volume over value when it comes to pregnancy in the United States.

Most obstetric practices are designed to process large numbers of patients—especially low-risk ones—so as to offset the high overhead inherent in contemporary American obstetrics. Indeed, many obstetricians are adept at running large volumes of patients through their offices. But processing mothers isn't the same as serving them. The average American obstetrician allows precious little time for a mother's questions or concerns to be addressed, and even less for any meaningful discussion to occur. A study by Mary D. Peoples-Sheps at the University of North Carolina, for example, found that only about half of pregnant women received routine counseling regarding pregnancy and health behaviors.[22]

The difference between quantity and quality in prenatal care is like that between McDonald's and Spago—both serve food, but where would you prefer to dine? Most doctors are trained to treat disease, not to maintain health; and pregnancy isn't a disease. Medicalization of pregnancy creates the illusion that prenatal care can provide a simple remedy for potential problems and diverts our attention from the more difficult issues which surround prematurity, low birthweight, and infant mortality. How have we come to believe that a brief prenatal care visit can counteract the harmful effects of unhealthy home situations and counterproductive maternal behavior? For what transpires at many prenatal visits, mothers could phone in their health information and have similar pregnancy outcomes. Not surprisingly, the prenatal care industry has seized upon the idea of prenatal care by phone—expect to see more of it in the future. But few innovations in modern obstetrics are designed to allow more interaction between mothers and their obstetricians. Rather, they're designed so that obstetricians can extend themselves further, thereby handling ever more mothers and the revenues they generate. By placing more gadgets and ancillary personnel between him/her and the mother, the obstetrician has become the overseer rather than the provider of care. With the use of physician "extenders" (nurses, technicians, and a host of assistants), the obstetrician can effectively franchise him/herself across a community. Care can be provided in each of his/her offices without him/her actually having to be in attendance, leading to inevitable questions regarding the necessity of obstetricians for low-risk prenatal care at all. 9

The Problem

We may infer the effectiveness of any system of prenatal care from the resultant outcomes. Many techniques have been devised to evaluate pregnancy outcome, such as:

- miscarriage rate
- fetal anomaly rate
- cesarean delivery rate
- fetal death rate, and
- maternal death rate.

Some of these techniques are more meaningful assays than others. But of all the measurable parameters, there's nothing in contemporary obstetrics responsible for more neonatal death and disability among non-anomalous babies than premature birth.[23] Prematurity occurs in 8 to 10 percent of births in America but accounts for 75 percent of all perinatal deaths.[24] Indeed, compared to babies of normal birthweight, preterm babies have a fortyfold greater death rate.[25] Among those babies weighing less than 1,500 grams (3.3 lbs.) who are lucky enough to survive, mental retardation, cerebral palsy and seizure disorders are twenty-two times more likely to occur.[26]

Definitions

To address the complex issue of prematurity, it's necessary to understand commonly used obstetrical terms:

- *Prematurity* has classically been ascribed to any newborn with a birthweight less than 2,500 grams (5.5 lbs.).

- *Preterm* is used to describe a baby born prior to thirty-seven weeks gestation (259 days from the first day of the mother's last menstrual period).

10

Although doctors frequently interchange these terms, they are not synonymous. Prematurity relates to birthweight while preterm refers to gestational age. Historically, babies weighing less than 2,500 grams were assumed to be premature. While this is generally the case, a few term babies will also fall below this weight. Nevertheless, most equate a birthweight less than 2,500 grams with prematurity because it's sometimes impossible to accurately determine a baby's true gestational age.

- *Low birthweight* includes newborns, irrespective of gestational age, who weigh less than 2,500 grams at birth. The large majority of these babies are preterm.

Although it fails to distinguish preterm infants from those who are simply small for their gestational age, the rate of low-birthweight babies is the most commonly used outcome measure because:

- Low birthweight is the largest contributor to infant mortality and therefore provides a surrogate measure of prematurity.
- Birthweight is easily quantifiable and readily available on birth certificates.

In simplest terms, this book addresses the issue of babies who are too small because they are too young. The imprecision and overlapping meanings of obstetrical terms may dishearten those with an interest in the topic—to avoid bogging-down in undue detail, this book will sacrifice a degree of precision and use the terms "preterm" and "premature" synonymously, unless otherwise specified. Likewise, "low birthweight" will generally be used to imply prematurity with full acknowledgment that some low-birthweight babies are small for reasons other than prematurity.

Other important terms for students of prenatal care relate to the different phases of gestation:

- *Prenatal (antenatal) period.* The period of time prior to delivery.
- *Neonatal period.* The first twenty-eight days of a baby's life. A child

during this period may be referred to as a neonate or newborn. A neonatologist is a pediatrician with special training and expertise in the care of premature or sick newborns.

- *Perinatal period.* The time span from the twenty-first week of gestation through the first twenty-eight days of life. In general, the term perinatal is used synonymously (but incorrectly) with the term prenatal. A perinatologist is an obstetrician/gynecologist with special training and expertise in the care of complicated pregnancies and maternal conditions. Perinatologists are sometimes called maternal-fetal or high-risk specialists.

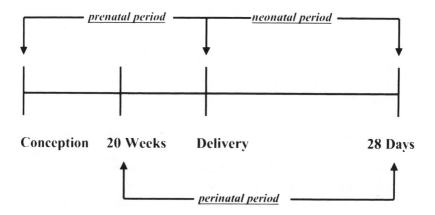

For the premature baby, time in the neonatal intensive care unit constitutes lifesaving misery. The child is pinioned in its incubator by a breathing tube and by catheters that course into its heart from a portal of entry in its navel. Twenty-four hours a day, the "preemie" is subjected to the sensory overload of a bright, painful place. Perpetually out of breath and out of touch from its mother, the child teeters on the brink for days or even weeks, so fragile that the simple act of feeding can sometimes trigger a life-threatening crisis as the child expends its tiny energy reserves on digestion. The slightest provocation can cause a debilitating or fatal stroke as delicate blood vessels throughout its brain rupture and bleed. Neonatal intensive care is the single most expensive service in our nation's healthcare system. The economic impact that this has is enormous, with daily charges sometimes exceeding $3,000 for a single preemie.[27]

Moreover:

12

- Preterm babies require five million days of in-hospital care annually.[28]
- On average, $30,000 to $150,000 (in 1996 dollars) are spent to graduate a single sick newborn from the intensive care unit.[29, 30]
- Babies with birthweights less than 1,000 grams (2.2 lbs.) cost an average of $210,000 (in 1996 dollars).[31, 32]
- Lifetime custodial care may be as high as $675,000 per child (in 1996 dollars).[33, 34]

Reprinted with permission from the American College of Obstetricians and Gynecologists from *Obstetrics and Gynecology* 76, Number 15(1990)55.

According to Dr. John C. Morrison at the University of Mississippi, "The proportionate costs of cancer, myocardial infarction, [kidney] transplants, etc. have not risen nearly as dramatically as those for neonatal intensive care."[35]

In the United States, roughly 400,000 preterm babies are born annually—that is, 45 per hour. And because prematurity is more frequently associated with low socioeconomic status, its economic burden is borne heavily by public sources of funding such as Medicaid, thereby exacting a considerable toll on society as a whole.[36] Prematurity is an emotionally devastating experience for everyone involved. For example, divorce rates are higher for families with premature babies (especially impaired ones). Thus, the effectiveness of American prenatal care will be reflected in its prematurity rate—and it's with this measuring stick that we can see how far behind the rest of the industrialized world we've fallen.

Consider this:

- In 1990, the United States' low birthweight rate ranked thirty-first among developed nations.[37] Despite enormous expenditures for prenatal care, the percentage of low-birthweight babies born in the United States is not much different than it was in the 1940s.[38] By comparison, Japan and Sweden boast premature delivery rates that are one-half of that in America.[39] Not only has the incidence of prematurity failed to decline in the United States, it is on the rise.
- Twenty-two industrialized nations had infant mortality rates that were lower than that of the United States in 1996:[40]

	Deaths per 1,000 Births
Singapore	3.8
Japan	3.8
Finland	4.0
Sweden	4.0
Norway	4.0
Hong Kong	4.0
Switzerland	4.7
Spain	4.7
France	4.9
Germany	5.0
Austria	5.1
Ireland	5.5
Belgium	5.6
Canada	5.6
Denmark	5.7
Netherlands	5.7
Australia	5.8
Italy	6.0
Czech Republic	6.0
United Kingdom	6.1
New Zealand	6.7
Portugal	6.9
United States	7.3

Reprinted by permission of *Pediatrics*, from B. Guyer, J. A. Martin, M. F. MacDorman, R. N. Anderson, D. M. Strobino. "Annual Summary of Vital Statistics—1996." *Pediatrics* 100 (1997)905.

Moreover, Sweden, the country with one of the world's lowest infant mortality rates, has per-capita health expenditures which are perennially a fraction of those in the United States.[41] In 1970, 1980 and 1993, for example, Swedish versus American expenditures (in U.S. dollars) were 271 versus 346, 855 versus 1068, and 1266 versus 3299, respectively. A number of other nations with infant mortality rates below that of the United States (including Canada, Denmark, France, Germany, Italy, Japan, the Netherlands, and the United Kingdom) also have had lower per-capita health expenditures from 1970 through 1993.[42]

Counterpoint

It might be argued that the United States' poor international standing is due in part to differences in reporting practices around the world. As a result, our

14 nation's infant mortality rate may be artificially high relative to other industrialized countries. At least eighty nations accept the official World Health Organization definition of a live birth (any newborn exhibiting any sign of life).[43] But it's been suggested that some governments routinely report some live births as stillbirths, thereby understating their infant mortality rates.[44] In France, for example, registration of birth is allowed to occur up to forty-eight hours after delivery. Liveborn infants who die prior to registration may be recorded as stillbirths.[45–47] In Japan, recent laws stipulate that only babies older than twenty-two weeks gestation (compared to twenty weeks in the United States) should be considered live births.[48] Japanese infants younger than twenty-two weeks (i.e., those with no hope of survival due to extreme prematurity) will elude classification as infant deaths. According to Benjamin P. Sachs at Harvard University, "Infant mortality provides a poor comparative measure of reproductive outcome because there are enormous regional and international differences in clinical practices and in the way live births are classified."[49]

When international infant mortality rates from 1992 are adjusted so as to exclude infant deaths of those weighing less than 1,000 grams (2.2 lbs.) and those with lethal congenital anomalies, our nation's relative standing is less discouraging:[50]

	Infant Mortality Rate*	Adjusted Rate*
England and Wales	7.7	4.9
France	7.4	4.7
Japan	4.4	4.0
United States	10.1	4.5

* per 1,000 live births
Reprinted with permission from the American College of Obstetricians and Gynecologists from *Obstetrics and Gynecology*. 85 (1995)941.

In 1994, 22 countries had infant mortality rates ranging from 4.2 deaths per 1,000 births (Japan) to 8.0 per 1,000 (United States)—dramatic improvements over 1930 infant mortality rates of 124.0 and 60.0, respectively, for these two nations.[51]

Compensating for possible underreporting of live births by excluding all babies that succumb in the first hour of life (as some countries reportedly do) would have reduced the United States' infant mortality rate to roughly 7 per 1,000 live births, thereby improving our international standing.

Rebuttal

Even if tinkering with calculations of our infant mortality rate were accept-   **15**
able, America's "revised" infant mortality rate would only have raised our
1994 international standing from twenty-second to seventeenth, according
to Dr. Myron E. Wegman at the University of Michigan. Furthermore, Dr.
Bernard Guyer of Johns Hopkins University notes, "Even if reporting con-
ventions were similar, it is likely that the U.S. rate would still remain higher
than the rate for many other countries because of the high percentage of
low-birthweight, particularly very low birthweight, births that occur in this
country relative to other developed countries."[52]

If we shift from infant mortality to the issue of low birthweight as a measuring stick, we still have an imperfect tool for gauging the effectiveness of
prenatal care, but such a shift allows us to focus solely on factors in the prenatal period. By this measure, the United States still lags behind most of the
industrialized world. According to the Annual Survey of Vital Statistics
which is published in the journal *Pediatrics*, the percentage of low-birthweight American infants born in 1997 was the highest since 1973, despite
the fact that the percentage of mothers who began prenatal care in the first
trimester rose to 82.5 percent and the percentage with late or no care fell to
4 percent.[53]

Prematurity isn't the only problem that can occur during pregnancy. But
in terms of infant mortality, there's nothing worse. Even so, it's worth examining the effect that prenatal care has on other pregnancy complications
because it illustrates our overconfidence in the present system:

Birth Defects. Even under ideal conditions, 2–3 percent of all pregnancies
will be complicated by birth defects, a statistic that's remained constant for
generations.[54] Birth defects generally arise during the early weeks of gestation, a time when many mothers don't even know they're with child. Beyond
this point, fetal anomalies generally cannot occur.[55] Prenatal care has nothing to do with it, whether it's provided by obstetricians, nurse-midwives, or
not at all. To be fair, some steps can be taken to reduce the occurrence of
certain birth defects. Dietary supplementation with the vitamin known as
folic acid (also called folate) may reduce some types of brain and spinal cord
defects, for example.[56, 57] Other measures include avoidance of certain drugs
or activities known to induce fetal anomalies. But for these regimens to be
most effective, they must be initiated before conception. For example, pregnancies must be planned so that folic acid supplementation can be properly

16

timed. No small amount of maternal self-control is necessary so that unhealthful activities are curtailed, something that routine American prenatal care has a poor track record at fostering. Besides, these regimens don't require the supervision of obstetricians. Folic acid, for example, can be purchased in any grocery store. Once a birth defect does occur, it can only rarely be fixed in utero. And for those that can be remedied or for those that require special care during pregnancy, maternal-fetal specialists are usually the care providers. In general, the best that prenatal care can offer when it comes to birth defects is the hope of early detection so that the family can choose whether or not to continue with the pregnancy. But the misuse of prenatal ultrasound described in later chapters raises serious questions about the ability of routine prenatal care to detect such problems.

Maternal Death. Prenatal care is frequently portrayed as an effective tool for reducing the incidence of maternal death. But the reality is that most maternal deaths occur during labor or the postpartum period from conditions that aren't influenced by prenatal care. Although the maternal death rate has fallen over the course of the twentieth century, it has come via general improvements in public health and specific advancements in transfusion science, surgical technology, and the development of antibiotics. Moreover, the frequency of maternal death (0.1 percent) is several orders of magnitude less than that of prematurity.[58] Indeed, the death of a healthy mother is almost unheard of in contemporary obstetrics. Yet it's the terrifying image of a pregnancy-related death which lingers in the minds of mothers and the rhetoric of advocates, thereby overshadowing the paltry evidence that prenatal care itself averts such uncommon events. Notwithstanding, maternal mortality in the United States increased in 1996 (the most recent year for which data is available) to 7.6 deaths per 100,000 live births, a death rate which is worse than twenty other nations around the world.[59]

Chromosomal Abnormalities. The issue of fetal chromosomal abnormalities is similar to that of birth defects. Indeed, many birth defects are caused by underlying genetic problems. But unlike certain types of birth defects, there's nothing we can do to reduce the incidence of chromosomal abnormalities or to remedy them when they occur. A baby either has chromosomal abnormalities or it doesn't. Moreover, a given baby's genetic make-up is established at the moment of conception and is unalterable thereafter. For mothers whose babies are at risk for chromosomal abnormalities, genetic counseling and testing is appropriate. But certain points must be made about this aspect of prenatal care. First, genetic counseling and testing do not reduce the frequency of genetic abnormalities, they only allow them to be identified so that parents can make informed choices about whether or not to continue with their pregnancies. Second, genetic counseling and testing aren't always provided by obstetricians. Indeed, a study by Dr. Louise Wilkins-Haug at Harvard Medical School surveyed obstetricians around the nation, finding that fewer than half performed invasive diagnostic procedures such as genetic amniocentesis.[60] Dr. Wilkins-Haug also found that one in three obstetricians offered no counseling to their patients for even the most commonly encountered genetic problems such as Down syndrome or neural tube defects; fewer than half were able to assess mothers' risks for (or to identify the proper diagnostic tests for) the most common ethnic group/race-specific maladies such as cystic fibrosis, Tay-Sachs disease, or sickle cell disease. Moreover, fewer than one in three obstetricians in the survey were able to provide their patients with educational materials for these disorders. Most obstetricians must refer their patients to "specialists" for genetic issues if questions arise. To make matters worse, a sizable portion of obstetricians, having already referred their patients out for genetic testing, choose not to dirty their hands by performing abortions on those wishing to terminate their genetically abnormal fetuses. Instead, their patients are frequently referred to yet another "specialist" to perform the deed so as to avoid the political heat that sometimes accompanies abortion.

Preeclampsia. Preeclampsia is a mysterious disease. Characterized by hypertension, temporary kidney malfunction, and sometimes seizures, preeclampsia only occurs in pregnant women; following childbirth, it vanishes. It's a dreaded pregnancy complication that can kill or injure mothers and their babies. As mentioned earlier, the entire system of prenatal care that American mothers have inherited has been shaped in large measure by our historical obsession with preeclampsia. The general frequency of prenatal care visits and the activities that persist to this day during a routine prenatal examination are geared towards the detection of this disease. But there's one problem with this strategy: prenatal care does nothing to reduce the occurrence of preeclampsia. In fact, its incidence is no different now than it's ever been. Like so many other pregnancy complications, preeclampsia either occurs or it doesn't. And until it does, there's little that obstetricians or midwives can do about it. Even when preeclampsia does develop, there's no cure except delivery. Despite all of our advancements, the best we can do is buy time before proceeding with delivery, thereby allowing more time for fetal growth to occur.

18

Medical Complications. A small proportion of mothers have medical problems that complicate their pregnancies. Virtually any illness can strike, from diabetes to cancer and from lupus to AIDS. To the extent that disease can harm mothers, it can also adversely affect their babies. Prior to the advent of insulin, for example, successful pregnancies were almost unheard of among diabetics. For many ill mothers today, medical care can result in better outcomes. This is the small province where intensively medicalized prenatal care can spell the difference between life and death. And it's upon this small subset of mothers that obstetricians should focus their efforts. Unfortunately, it's sick patients that many obstetricians most want to avoid, preferring instead to see healthy, low-maintenance mothers and referring out the more taxing cases. But in so doing, obstetricians forfeit their role in the very aspect of prenatal care that, at least in theory, separates them from midwives, general practitioners, and family physicians.

Counterpoint

Since 1979, causes of death in the United States have been classified according to the International Classification of Diseases.[61] Using this as a guide, we can see how the outcomes of America's babies have improved:[62]

Rank Cause of Infant Mortality Decrease Since 1979 (%)	
1. Congenital anomalies	35.4
2. Disorders relating to short gestation/low birthweight	5.3
3. Sudden Infant Death Syndrome (SIDS)	50.9
4. Respiratory Distress Syndrome (RDS)	77.7
5. Maternal complications of pregnancy	33.2
6. Complications of placenta, cord, membranes	18.0
7. Infections specific to the perinatal period	31.0
8. Accidents	37.5
9. Intrauterine hypoxia and birth asphyxia	70.7
10. Pneumonia, influenza	68.4

Reprinted by permission of *Pediatrics*, from B. Guyer, J. A. Martin, M. F. MacDorman, R. N. Anderson, D. M. Strobino. "Annual Summary of Vital Statistics—1996." *Pediatrics* 100(1997)905.

The ten leading causes of infant death in the United States have undergone an overall decrease of 45.6 percent between 1979 and 1997. Indeed, the infant mortality rate for the United States in 1997 was 7.1 deaths per 1,000 **19** live births, the lowest ever recorded in this nation.

Rebuttal

Despite the drop in infant mortality, our prenatal care is not necessarily improving. Infant mortality is an imperfect measure of prenatal care's efficacy because there are a number of postpartum factors, such as neonatal care, that influence it. Clearly, events in the prenatal period may affect the infant mortality rate, but post-delivery factors cloud the issue somewhat. Let's look at each of the top ten causes of infant death individually to illustrate the point:

1. *Anomalies.* As mentioned earlier, birth defects either happen or they don't. By the time that many mothers even realize they're pregnant, the vulnerable period for fetal anomalies has come and gone. Thus, while prenatal care affords the opportunity to identify fetal defects, it doesn't actually reduce their frequency of occurrence. The decrease in infant mortality as a result of congenital anomalies is due in large part to two factors: First, many anomalous babies are aborted by their mothers, and thus the number of abnormal babies that actually reach infancy is reduced. In effect, abortion merely shifts their deaths to an earlier point in time. Second, some infants are able to survive with congenital anomalies, not because of prenatal care, but because of advancements in neonatal and pediatric therapies.

2. *Prematurity/Low Birthweight.* Babies from this category account for a large share of neonatal and infant deaths, and prenatal care has had minimal effect in preventing this problem. Indeed, of the top ten killers of infants, this category has experienced by far the smallest decrease since 1979. Moreover, the small decrease in infant mortality within this category was due in large part to neonatal therapeutic advancements. As Dr. Bernard Guyer, the author/compiler of the U.S.'s Annual Survey of Vital Statistics (1996), points out, "Low birthweight and preterm delivery [are] one of the most significant challenges facing the medical professional in the next decade."[63]

3. *Sudden Infant Death Syndrome (SIDS).* SIDS rates have fallen 38 percent since 1992 when the American Academy of Pediatrics issued a

recommendation to reduce SIDS by placing infants on their backs or sides to sleep.[64] Obviously, this preventative recommendation falls outside the realm of obstetrics, and the decrease in SIDS deaths cannot be attributed to prenatal care.

4. Respiratory Distress Syndrome (RDS). RDS is a problem found almost exclusively among premature babies. Thus, high RDS rates reflect our nation's problem with preterm birth. Infant mortality rates from RDS have fallen over 60 percent since 1989 when new neonatal treatments became available, not from advancements in prenatal care.

5. Maternal Complications. These constitute high-risk pregnancies. In general and increasingly, these pregnancies are attended to outside of the arena of "routine" prenatal care. Many times, treatment of certain maternal complications requires the doctor to deliver a sick mother's baby prematurely. Thus, the actual survival of the child is dependent upon neonatal care rather than prenatal care.

6. Placenta, Umbilical Cord, Membranes. Patients with problems in these areas also fall into the "high-risk" pregnancy category. Indeed, the artificial categorization regarding causes of infant mortality tend to ignore the overlap of certain complications which occur naturally. The comments provided under category 5 ("maternal complications") also apply here. Prenatal care does not reduce the occurrence of these spontaneously occurring natural problems.

7. Infections Specific to the Perinatal Period. The bulk of these infections occurs when the fetal membranes or "bag of waters" rupture, thereby allowing germs access to the intrauterine cavity and fetus. Preterm rupture of the membranes is a common precursor to preterm labor and delivery. Thus, preterm rupture could be considered a subgroup of prematurity/low birthweight. Advancements in antibiotic treatments and neonatal care are the primary reason for the improved survival rates of these babies. Available evidence does not demonstrate that prenatal care reduces the incidence of premature rupture of the fetal membranes.

8. Accidents. Obviously, prenatal care cannot prevent accidents from occurring.

20

9. Hypoxia/Asphyxia. Severe asphyxia can sometimes be associated with cerebral palsy and/or death. Fetal hypoxia/asphyxia which occurs during childbirth is unrelated to prenatal care; the majority of compromised babies, however, are silently damaged during the prenatal period. Indeed, the condition is usually unanticipated by mother and doctor. Routine prenatal care has not reduced the overall incidence of cerebral palsy in the United States, despite the fact that infant mortality attributable to hypoxia/asphyxia has fallen.[65] In part, survival has increased within this group as a result of the ever-improving resuscitative skills of neonatologists and pediatricians.   **21**

10. Pneumonia and Influenza. Diseases such as these are not prevented by prenatal care.

Prenatal Care Doesn't Prevent Prematurity

Most interventions designed to prevent preterm birth do not work, and the few that do . . . are not universally effective and are applicable to only a small percentage of women at risk for preterm birth.[66]
—Robert L. Goldenberg, M.D., University of Alabama

When it comes to healthy individuals, it's frequently difficult to know whether certain medical regimens are really providing benefit or whether it's the patients' vigor which actually makes the difference. Clearly, there are some who've been helped by prenatal care. But despite many advances in obstetrics, there have been no appreciable reductions in America's prematurity rate since the days when cars had tailfins. At a large inner-city medical center in Cleveland, for example, the proportion of mothers delivering low-birthweight babies actually increased between 1975 and 1992.[67] A similar trend occurred in Arizona between 1980 and 1995.[68, 69] Over the decade of the '80s and thus far into the '90s, Arizona women who received an adequate number of prenatal care visits have accounted for an increasing proportion of low-birthweight babies. Nationwide, the story is disappointingly similar to that noted in Cleveland and Arizona. In fact, analysis of national statistics reveals that the number of American mothers who receive an inadequate number of prenatal care visits fell steadily over the '80s and '90s, yet the percentage of American women delivering low-birthweight babies rose during the same period.

Certainly, facts like these force us to question whether contemporary American prenatal care is doing anything to counteract prematurity. To an

22 objective, rational scientist, the quandary would suggest that there's something wrong with American prenatal care. But, to the true believers, it infers nothing of the sort. Rather, our steadily worsening prematurity rate is taken as a mandate to provide even more prenatal care to our mothers.

Counterpoint

One could argue that prematurity and low-birthweight statistics are misleading because they ignore the fact that we are now delaying deliveries of many previable fetuses until they are sufficiently strong to survive outside of the womb.[70] To the same extent that we can prevent a thirty-five-week baby from delivering until thirty-seven weeks (i.e., term), we can also delay delivery of a twenty-two-week fetus (100 percent mortality rate) until twenty-four weeks (35–50 percent mortality). Thus, the net effect of our efforts has not been a reduced incidence of preterm birth and low birthweight but a reduced incidence of death by "frameshifting" the gestational age composition of premature/low-birthweight babies.

Rebuttal

Some low-birthweight babies are sicker and require more care than others. While a decrease in the number of babies at the upper end of the low-birthweight category (1,500–2,499 grams—the group that accounts for 83 percent of all low-birthweight babies) influences the overall low-birthweight rate, it ignores the fact that a disproportionate share of expenses arise from very low-birthweight (less than 1,500 grams) babies.[71] Moreover, those tiniest of babies who just scrape across the viability line bare the brunt of prematurity's ravages: permanent disability is concentrated among babies at the lowest end of the birthweight spectrum. Although some babies do eventually triumph over extreme prematurity, for too many it's a Pyrrhic victory. Very low-birthweight babies comprise only 1 percent of all births yet account for 46 percent of infant deaths.[72] Thus, while our "frameshift" has supposedly produced more term or near-term babies, it has also yielded a large supply of very low birthweight babies.

According to 1996 statistics, the proportion of very low-birthweight babies among white mothers was at its highest level since 1970.[73] Among mothers in the African-American community, the very low-birthweight rate has not budged since the late 1980s. Therefore, for every dollar purportedly saved when a preterm baby's delivery is delayed until term, an even greater amount is spent to care for the very low-birthweight child who's been nudged across the viability line: the initial medical costs for infants in the 1,500- to 1,999-gram range are roughly ten times greater than for normal births. To make matters worse, "frameshift" hasn't led to static low-birthweight rates as is sometimes claimed; 1996 and 1997 data demonstrates that not only has our very low-birthweight rate increased, the overall low-birthweight rate is climbing too, a fact which echoes throughout this chapter.

It's also important to note that much of the "frameshift" phenomenon mentioned above (especially among those babies at the lower end of the low-birthweight spectrum) is a result of intensive medical care which generally requires hospitalization, intravenous medications, and a host of aggressive medical interventions. Moreover, such intensive care is something that's initiated only after preterm labor has started. Except for the fact that this care is rendered prenatally, it bears little resemblance to what we consider routine prenatal care to be. In the final analysis, the one constant is that routine prenatal care does not prevent the onset of preterm labor.

An Ounce of Prevention

Effective preventive measures are essentially unavailable, largely because we do not know how to predict the problem with enough certainty to warrant enrolling patients in a trial of preventive approaches.[74]
　　　　　　　　　　—Robert K. Creasy, M.D., University of San Diego

Prenatal care has been portrayed as a form of preventive medicine. Although this characterization might seem reasonable, prematurity prevention programs have been disappointing. None have worked on a widespread or prolonged basis. Yet it's the perception of prenatal care as the quintessence of preventive medicine that places it at the vanguard of women's healthcare issues. A host of tests developed by the world's leading obstetric and pediatric authorities have attempted to identify mothers at risk for prematurity, but none have met with consistent or widespread success because:

24

- The tests are imperfect and have limited predictive value.
- A considerable number of mothers with no apparent risk nevertheless develop pregnancy-related complications.
- For many with identifiable risk factors, little can be done to modify them.

According to Dr. Greg R. Alexander of the University of Alabama, "The findings of the multi-centered preterm prevention trials in the United States suggest that the approaches taken there have failed. Indeed, rates of preterm birth in the United States appear to be increasing in spite of these and other community-wide efforts."[75] Likewise, K. Danbe of Kaiser-Permanente in California laments, "Current tools to predict increased risk for preterm delivery . . . have shown limited value for improving outcome."[76]

Dr. William E. Roberts at the University of Mississippi reviewed data gleaned from over 17,000 mothers felt to be at high risk for preterm labor based on the presence of four risk factors (prior history of preterm labor, multiple gestations, uterine abnormalities, and/or cervical abnormalities) that have been most consistently associated with prematurity.[77] Dr. Roberts found that only 40 percent of these mothers experienced preterm labor. Contemporary American obstetrics is based upon the concept of prevention—an expensive and ineffective undertaking. Nowadays, obstetric breakthroughs progress from discovery to entitlement without regard to efficacy. A 1995 publication on preterm labor from the American College of Obstetricians and Gynecologists—the governing body of American obstetricians—concedes, "Despite a great deal of research and the introduction of new diagnostic and therapeutic technologies, there has been little or no improvement in outcome. Although there are many different therapies available, there is great controversy over their effectiveness in the prevention of prematurity and the management of patients in preterm labor."[78] But there is little controversy that risk-factor analysis for prematurity has produced an increase in intervention with techniques of uncertain or unproven effectiveness. Lost in the discussion, however, is the fact that the strongest predictor of prematurity is a history of preterm delivery with a previous pregnancy. But since roughly half of preterm births occur in women having their first child, risk-scoring systems are severely handicapped when it comes to this group of mothers.[79]

More Is Less

Given the long-held mindset that prenatal care is the solution to prematu-   **25**
rity, it might seem perfectly reasonable to assume that more intensive prenatal care would produce even better results. However, these assumptions
wither under the scrutiny of objective research. Among the many published
reports of enhanced prenatal care, all but the original two have utterly failed
to reduce the rate of prematurity.[80–94]

In 1982, Ms. M. A. Herron conducted a year-long study of women at
high risk for preterm labor who participated in a prematurity prevention
program at the University of California in San Francisco.[95] The mothers
were instructed in the detection of the early signs of preterm labor and
were followed weekly in a special prenatal clinic. Herron's data indicated
that there was a statistically significant decrease in the incidence of preterm delivery among program participants. Likewise, a twelve-year study
by Dr. E. Papiernik in Haguenau, France, attributed a steady, significant
decrease in the preterm birth rate to an interventive prematurity prevention program. However, Dr. Papiernik did not observe a reduction in prematurity among high-risk mothers, a phenomenon that would repeat itself
in subsequent studies.

Of special concern was the fact that no improvement was observed among
mothers with previous preterm deliveries. For these women, the prematurity
rate remained static throughout the twelve-year span of Dr. Papiernik's
study. Moreover, reduced rates of prematurity were not unique to mothers
who participated in the study: fewer preterm births were also noted across
all of France during the twelve-year period, raising questions about the utility of the prematurity prevention program.[96] Encouraged by these reports
nonetheless, studies seeking to confirm the benefits of intensive, interventive
prenatal programs followed. While the specific content of interventive programs varied somewhat, all were similar in that they focused on women determined to be at high risk for prematurity. Aggressive measures were taken
to prolong their pregnancies. All but one program took measures to educate
mothers about the signs and symptoms of preterm labor. All but a few placed
high-risk patients into specialized clinics where mothers were seen and examined more frequently than they would have been had they attended routine prenatal care clinics. Many utilized special personnel to give nutritional
advice, psychological, and emotional support, as well as substance abuse and
stress-reduction counseling. Although some interventive programs claimed
isolated successes at reducing the preterm delivery rate in certain subgroups,

the results have not been consistently duplicated or sustained by subsequent research. Thus, despite our best intentions and best efforts, we have not met with the success we had hoped for. According to Dr. Claudia Holzman of Michigan State University,

26

> Attempts to reduce the incidence of preterm delivery through the use of risk-scoring protocols, frequent cervical assessment, cervical cerclage, home monitoring of uterine contractions, tocolytic therapy, enhanced prenatal care and social support programs have by and large been unsuccessful. In fact, preterm delivery rates have been climbing steadily in the United States, from 9.4% to 10.7% in 1992.[97]

There is also considerable evidence that suggests that prenatal care—especially intensive interventive programs of care—is much less successful with indigent populations than with private patients. For example, Dr. Paul J. Meis at the Bowman Gray School of Medicine evaluated the effectiveness of a regional program for preventing preterm deliveries in northwestern North Carolina.[98] Like the great majority of interventive programs, the overall prematurity rate was not significantly reduced. However, a subpopulation of women with private health insurance did experience significant reductions in prematurity. Likewise, Dr. Saeid B. Amini analyzed births from eighteen consecutive years at Cleveland Medical Center.[99] Despite a significantly increased overall rate of preterm births during the eighteen-year period, for privately insured mothers, the mean gestational age increased by more than one week while the mean gestational age for indigent patients actually declined by a week. Thus, it seems that the highest risk group benefits the least from interventive programs designed to reduce prematurity. Closer scrutiny of M. A. Herron's pioneering study of prematurity prevention—one of the few studies that demonstrated any overall benefit from an interventive prenatal program—reveals that the mothers studied were essentially middle-class women, not the indigent or inner-city women frequently used in less successful projects. It would appear, therefore, that the success of a prematurity program will be strongly influenced by the characteristics of the patients included in the program.

Poor women generally fare less well because prenatal care can't compensate for the many problems that often complicate their lives. To a well-nourished, well-rested middle-class woman, prenatal care is like icing on the cake. But to a woman living in poverty, pregnancy can sometimes represent the last straw; and a series of pointless, ill-explained visits to an obstetrician will not likely counteract the morass of detrimental conditions which surround her twenty-four hours a day.

Despite the well-documented association between poor pregnancy out-   **27**
comes and maternal behaviors like smoking and substance abuse (risk factors more common among the poor), many doctors don't even bother
looking for them. After reviewing the prenatal records of nearly 1,000
doctors, for example, Dr. Mary D. Peoples-Sheps at the University of
North Carolina found that only 51 percent asked their patients about alcohol use, only 44 percent queried about drug use and only 59 percent
asked about smoking.[100] Dr. Peoples-Sheps' findings naturally beg the
question as to how prenatal care can favorably impact these problems if we
ignore them. When it comes to the home situations of American mothers,
doctors seem even less interested, despite the widely acknowledged influence of socioeconomic status on pregnant women. Peoples-Sheps found
that only 27 percent asked their patients about social problems, only 6
percent asked about financial stress, and only 19 percent offered education regarding prenatal nutrition. While doctors often consider voluntary
behaviors such as smoking and the home life of their patients to be outside of their official perview, time spent attending to and advising their patients about what they can do to improve their conditions and their health
would likely prove to have a beneficial impact.

Insufficient Knowledge

**Only when the factors underlying prematurity are completely understood
can any progress be made.**[101]

—Nicholson J. Eastman, M.D., 1947

One medical researcher recently characterized prematurity as the "largest
unsolved mystery in medicine." Indeed, we still have an incomplete understanding of prematurity despite assertions to the contrary in some
quarters. Undaunted, one newspaper columnist recently announced that
"doctors and healthcare providers can identify about 80 percent of
women likely to have low-birthweight or sick babies,"[102] while an Institute of Medicine publication went so far as to proclaim that "little will be
accomplished by further efforts to document the value of prenatal
care."[103] But theories regarding the cause and treatment of prematurity
based on incomplete or incorrect information are doomed to failure; over

the decades, hypotheses have come and gone. According to Dr. Claudia Holzman of Michigan State University, "Our knowledge of the natural history of this complex and probably multi-determined health state is very limited."[104] Dr. Holzman's comments are echoed by a growing number of prematurity researchers. For example, Dr. Greg R. Alexander of the University of Alabama summarized the proceedings of an international conference on preterm birth as follows: "It was stressed that we must be honest with policymakers and the public about what has actually been shown to work and concerns were voiced that previously overly optimistic endorsements of poorly tested interventions resulted in the widespread ineffective use of precious resources."[105]

A Problem of Perception

Any given controversy is decided not on the basis of the kind of evidence that is produced by biomedical research . . . rather its status will depend on how well it fits with the sociopolitical realities and the ideological belief system of its time and place.[106]

—Brigitte Jordan, anthropologist

It is possible that valid scientific evidence . . . may be obscured, suppressed and not fully evaluated if it is not in tune with our society's system of beliefs.[107]

—Dr. John H. Kennell, Case Western University

Throughout history, pregnancy has been venerated as the acme of femininity. It's an important event, an integral part of the birth-marriage-death triad at the center of most cultures. In Western society, pregnant women are viewed as fetal surrogates: what's done to the mother is ultimately done to her child. The two exist concentrically. As gestational vessels, mothers have come to represent the rind of deeper, more precious fruit. In America, prenatal care is the icon of maternity, a symbol of our regard for the nearborn. For almost one hundred years, ritualized prenatal care has been accepted as an article of faith in the United States, having long ago become part of our cultural lore and a province of medicine. Our system is founded on the best of intentions. But does it make a difference? Unlike the maladies that we conquered earlier this century, prematurity doesn't maim or kill mothers. But one thing that history has shown us is that prematurity can be triggered by any number of events, many of which defy straightforward medical explanations.

Much of what passes for prenatal care in this country is unduly expensive, unnecessarily high-tech, and serves no beneficial purpose, consisting of little more than a string of pointless, largely ceremonial clinic visits which infrequently avert the conditions we most want our babies to avoid. The problem is that we have oversimplified a complex issue that's received scant attention and even less objective analysis. Spurred by the impressive reduction in maternal and infant mortality rates that it appeared to produce earlier this century, we have advised all pregnant women to seek medical care. Public expenditures for prenatal care in the United States have been rationalized with windy assertions that it's an effective, cost-saving endeavor. However, the current support for prenatal care in this nation is more politically than scientifically based—but apparently, this is permissible when the cause is perceived to be a noble one.

Overview

The conventional wisdom that prenatal care is crucial to the well-being of mothers and their babies is incongruent with the findings of published medical research and our nation's experience over the last half-century. Thus, it's somewhat surprising that there are so few books that question its utility. The most recent rebuke of things obstetric is Jessica Mitford's book, *The American Way of Birth*.[108] But the late Ms. Mitford focuses almost exclusively on the labor process, leaving the issue of prenatal care unscathed. Therefore, *Expecting Trouble* explores new territory, and it does so by asking the question, What's the evidence? Within this context, there are certain aspects of prenatal care which *Expecting Trouble* will investigate:

The Historical, Political, and Scientific Basis of Prenatal Care (chapter 2). Prenatal care is frequently cited as one of the genuinely successful examples of preventive medicine. From the outset, prenatal care has been considered a cost-effective endeavor, a notion that's gone largely unchallenged. But what of the accuracy of the medical research that touts its economic utility? A close analysis of this research reveals a variety of flaws and unsupported assumptions, demonstrating the fallaciousness of cost-savings arguments. The administrative overgrowth and the bureaucracy that permeate our prenatal care system are currently burgeoning. Our system emphasizes self-preservation rather than quality of care, as specific examples make clear. Five additional examples demonstrate how mainstream American prenatal care practices have been widely accepted as standards of care despite a dearth of supporting scientific evidence regarding their effectiveness.

Maldistribution of Prenatal Resources (chapter 3). Increasingly, hospitals and doctors tend to retain high-risk mothers and babies for whom they have inadequate facilities. Research shows that newborn babies may be dying needlessly because sick mothers and babies are not being transferred to regional centers of excellence. In chapter 3, the assumption that obstetricians care for the most difficult cases is put to the test. Furthermore, as a number of studies from across the nation show, liberalized access to prenatal care does not necessarily increase maternal enrollment in prenatal clinics or improve outcomes. As a final case suggests, the movement to classify obstetrician/gynecologists as primary healthcare providers for women is clearly a step in the wrong direction.

Undue Medicalization of Pregnancy (chapter 4). Too often, pregnancy is wrongly perceived as a disease. The "medicalization" of pregnancy makes prenatal care more costly and may actually increase the risk of malpractice litigation. The medicalization of pregnancy doesn't necessarily improve pregnancy outcomes. As a number of studies demonstrate, the pregnancy outcomes among mothers receiving care from nurse-midwives and the outcomes of those cared for by obstetricians are equivalent.

Unwarranted or Misplaced Malpractice Litigation (chapter 4). A brief historical review of medical malpractice litigation in this country reveals that malpractice litigation has produced few, if any, real improvements in women's health. Several examples suggest that women may actually be worse off as a result of undue malpractice claims. After tracing the root causes of malpractice claims, chapter 4 offers solutions to the malpractice problem which ensure justice for genuine malpractice victims.

Avaricious Health Insurers (chapter 4). In addition to the objectives outlined above, the book also discusses the implications of managed care and demonstrates how managed care is forcing physicians to choose between their own economic well-being and the well-being of their patients.

Mothers Themselves (chapter 5). Central to the issue of prenatal care is the mother and her fetus. Research shows that mothers themselves may affect pregnancy outcomes to a greater degree than do their obstetricians. In chapter 5, the interplay of marital status, socioeconomic status, and race is discussed, and the influence of pregnancy wantedness is explored.

31

What We Can Do about It: Step One

There's much to be done if we're to improve American pregnancies. But the first thing we must do is change our mindset. We must look beyond the soft archetypal images that pregnancy conjures and allow for the possibility that all is not well. Indeed, a healthy dose of skepticism is just what the doctor ordered.

Recently, I was listening to a radio program which featured a popular public figure. Over the course of the interview, the guest presented a well-reasoned argument against affirmative action policies. The host of the show elucidated an equally splendid defense. No assumption was left unexamined; no claims were made without supporting evidence. Point by point, the two sparred in a most impressive fashion, raising some issues that I'd never previously considered and debunking others I'd long thought to be established fact. Eventually, the issue of healthcare—specifically, prenatal care—entered the discussion. Without hesitation, the two concurred that the lack of prenatal care among our "underclasses" was a contributor to the perpetuation of the poor's plight. I imagined the two pundits nodding in unison, having finally reached agreement on something. But unfortunately, when it comes to the most sacred of well-intended institutions, even critical thinkers let their guard down, trusting in prenatal care not only to improve the health of American babies but as a tool for social change. Instead, let's agree from the start upon the common goal of healthier babies and at the same time make room in the discussion for heretics. And let's acknowledge that the last four decades of standard, traditional maternity care hasn't seen a reduction in America's rate of prematurity or cerebral palsy.

As parents, let's stop spending money and effort where it isn't needed and focus on areas where it is. Let's question what (and whom) we haven't questioned before. Let's acknowledge a popular misconception and demand truth in advertising when it comes to the care we receive. As doctors, we must allow for the possibility that prenatal care as we provide it is probably not the vehicle that will help us arrive at our common goal. But let's also allow for the possibility that part of the answer to the problem of American pregnancies is already available to us, even if we don't like its implications. Searching for the answers to the problem of prenatal care, *Expecting Trouble* will elucidate the following claims:

32

- By the time that many American pregnancies are conceived, it's already too late to favorably impact their outcomes.
- Prenatal care as we know it provides benefits which have been overstated for the majority of our mothers.
- Prenatal care persists in the manner that it does in America because of the economic and political benefits it affords its supporters.
- Effective prenatal care is not a tool for social change, it's a reflection of social change.

2. The Basis of Prenatal Care

It is fair to say that most interventions designed to prevent preterm birth do not work. The few that do . . . have not been shown to be effective with all—or even most—women.[1]
                              —March of Dimes Research, Annual Report, 1998

Our fault lies with knowing that we have no treatment and not saying so. We must admit that the effective treatment of preterm labor remains only a goal.[2]
                    —Herbert F. Sandmire, M.D., University of Wisconsin

Although significant contributions to the field came from Britain, contemporary prenatal care is largely an American invention. The advent of organized care was credited by the great obstetrician Nicholson J. Eastman "with having done more to save mothers' lives than any other single factor," the most important advance in obstetrics of the preceding hundred years.[3] Indeed, nineteenth-century medical textbooks hardly mention the topic. Physicians of that era attended solely to laboring women and were sought during the prenatal period only if the mothers had seizures, hemorrhaged, or suffered other complications.

In 1901, English physician John W. Ballantyne persuaded the Royal Maternity Hospital to reserve a solitary bed for pregnant women.[4, 5] As a result of his insistence, the ensuing twenty years saw the expansion of his single maternity bed into a twenty-three-patient unit. By 1930, England had over 600 prenatal clinics. Simultaneously in the United States, the Instructive District Nursing Association of Boston was sending nurses into the homes of mothers enrolled in the Home Delivery Service. Each enrollee received at least one prenatal visit—by 1912, each mother received an average of three visits during her pregnancy.[6] At about the same time, the Boston Lying-In Hospital established the nation's first prenatal clinic.[7] For each mother at the clinic, a medical history was obtained and a physical examination performed which included blood pressure measurement and urinalysis. Each "patient" was instructed in hygiene and advised to return in one month—sooner if problems arose. When summoned, a nurse would visit the mother at home. The results were impressive. Following the establishment of organized prenatal care in New York City, for example, infant mortality rates fell by more than 70 percent.[8] Likewise, a study conducted in 1921 by the Metropolitan Life Insurance Company reported a reduction in the infant mortality rate by 29 percent and a reduction in maternal mortality by 21 percent among those who received care from New York City's Maternity Care Association.[9]

Birth of a Movement

Although prenatal care presently enjoys overwhelming popularity, it wasn't always so. Early initiatives designed to improve the lot of American mothers and infants were generally met with disinterest or recalcitrance. During the first decade of the twentieth century, for example, a bill to combat the nation's high infant mortality rate languished for years before it was signed into law by President Taft in 1912.[10] Six years later, Montana Congresswoman Jeanette Rankin introduced a bill for the "protection of maternity and infancy," proposing two million dollars to educate rural women regarding prenatal and infant care.[11] The *Illinois Medical Journal* derided the bill as: "A menace . . . another piece of destructive legislation sponsored by endocrine perverts, derailed menopausics and a lot of other men and women . . . working overtime . . . to destroy the country."[12] Strenuously opposed by organized medicine, Ms. Rankin's bill lapsed in committee until it was eventually resurrected by Senator Morris Sheppard and Representative Horace Towner in 1919.[13] Almost immediately, battle lines were drawn by competing special interest groups, with the American Medical Association in opposition and the Children's Bureau, the Department of Agriculture, and the American Federation of Labor in support. Bolstered by organized women's groups, the Sheppard-Towner Bill was finally passed in 1921 but with more modest appropriations than Ms. Rankin's original proposals. Eight years later, funding was discontinued.[14]

For Every Dollar Spent

In the tug-of-war between economic conservatism and social liberalism, the issue of cost-effectiveness has frequently been used to support or impugn many a government program. Likewise, the cost-savings argument has often been used to promote expansion of maternity care. In 1913, for example, the Boston Medical Surgical Journal calculated that the cost of prenatal care—$1.16 per mother—was economically feasible for any community with more than 500 deliveries annually.[15]

More recently, federal and state funding of prenatal care throughout the United States has been predicated on the assertion that it will save money over the long haul. By supposedly preventing the huge costs incurred by premature births, advocates declared that public spending for prenatal care would actually pay for itself. Since the 1970s, precise dollar projections of cost savings have convinced government policymakers that funding for the present system of maternity care is a prudent and worthwhile investment. You can imagine the popularity among politicians and taxpayers of any program that promises a return of $3.38 for every dollar spent.[16] Unfortunately, supporting evidence for the cost-effectiveness of prenatal care is less clear than one might guess, given the widespread acceptance of funding for it. The reality is that conclusions gleaned from most studies regarding the thriftiness of prenatal care contain fatal flaws. For example, when Dr. Jane Huntington of Group Health Cooperative in Seattle carefully reviewed over one hundred cost-effectiveness studies published in medical journals and government documents from 1975 through 1993, she found serious errors that may have resulted in sizable overestimations of cost savings attributable to prenatal care.[17]

In a similar vein, Dr. Marie C. McCormick of the Harvard School of Public Health analyzed more than seventy studies addressing economic issues related to prematurity, finding that economic information about the potential impact of intervention in or prevention of prematurity is "spotty and flawed."[18] Dr. McCormick concluded, "At this juncture, assessing the cost-effectiveness of potential interventions in changes in prevalence of prematurity might arrive at seriously flawed conclusions."

Dr. Wendy J. Smith of the University of Washington reviewed the cost-effectiveness claims of papers published in obstetrics and gynecology journals from 1990 through 1996.[19] Nearly one hundred articles were scrutinized for adherence to ten minimum standards for medical economic analyses. Only five conformed to all ten criteria. Dr. Smith concluded, "Even basic methodologic principles generally are not used in most economic analyses published in the obstetrics and gynecology literature." When it comes to the cost-effectiveness of prenatal care, the use of flawed data has important ramifications for policy decisions regarding the care of our nation's mothers.

Ensuring that pregnant women obtain prenatal care is far more complex and expensive than simply paying obstetricians' bills. Other issues that are almost never addressed by economists include the maldistribution of prenatal care providers, ensuring reliable transportation to and from prenatal clinics, meeting the various enrollment criteria of some prenatal clinics, and the lack of maternal motivation to seek care. But perhaps the greatest flaw in the cost-saving argument is the assumption that prenatal care reduces prematurity. It doesn't. And calculations that presuppose that it does are calculations which are erroneous.

36

Acknowledging the failure of intensive, specialized prenatal programs to reduce prematurity, some experts have retreated to the position that even "undetectable and seemingly insignificant reductions in low birthweight" may be cost-effective, a tactic that eliminates the need for prenatal care programs to actually demonstrate any objective, scientific medical benefits before they are embraced and funded.[20, 21] According to Dr. Huntington,

> The evidence that prenatal care pays for itself is simply not strong enough to merit the virtual certainty with which this claim has been espoused. . . . It has been commonplace but misleading to hold up prenatal care—especially the relatively inexpensive services provided to women at low risk—as the solution to the problems of children born in poverty. The current public perception of prenatal care oversimplifies the difficulties of delivering prenatal care to women who do not now receive it, oversimplifies the benefits of prenatal care and contributes to the medicalization of complex social problems. . . . Because the cost-savings argument has dominated the discussion, publicly funded prenatal care may be abandoned if it turns out not to pay for itself.[22]

According to Dr. James O. Mason, Assistant Secretary for Health and head of the Public Health Service in the early 1990s, the Administration's only new initiative (known as "Healthy Start") to reduce American's infant mortality was destined for success because: "We know enough right now to make a significant dent in the infant mortality rate and reach our goals for the year 2000."[23] Indeed, Dr. Mason concluded his address at a national conference on improving pregnancy outcomes by pronouncing that: "With good medicine for all, better outreach and best behavior, we can do as well as the Japanese." Healthy Start's specific goal was to reduce infant mortality by 50 percent over five years in American communities with extremely high infant mortality rates (at least 15.8 deaths per 1,000 live births) by concentrating on four things:

- Increased Medicaid enrollment and providers
- Promotion of family and a culture of character
- Enhanced content of prenatal care
- Targeted efforts to the local needs of communities with high infant mortality rates

In 1991, $25 million of funds were designated for the program, $171 million were earmarked in 1992 and a total of $500 million had been spent by 1995.[24] But a report on the actual impact of Healthy Start was squelched, according to the *Philadelphia Inquirer*, which claims that Healthy Start has had no effect on infant mortality in poor neighborhoods.[25] Findings by Mathematica Policy Research, Inc., a firm hired by the federal government to evaluate the progress at sixteen sites, were to be presented at a meeting of the American Public Health Association in 1997. But according to Mathematica spokesperson Joanne Pfleiderer, "The government chose to cancel our presentation at a late date. The abstract for this presentation was submitted almost a year ago."[26] According to the *Philadelphia Inquirer*, Mathematica found that Healthy Start had little impact on either infant mortality rates or the number of low-birthweight babies in Philadelphia and Chicago but was bound by government contract not to disclose the contents of its report. Although one can only surmise what the data shows, the federal government's behavior hardly suggests that the data is encouraging. But the government's behavior, moreover, illustrates the political investment that some have made in prenatal programs.

The political attractiveness of prenatal care is unmistakable. As with many politically popular policies, however, it's seldom challenged. Public support for prenatal care is now so widespread that proponents need only invoke moral rationales to further their cause. Demonstrations of efficacy aren't necessary, and, in consequence, some aspects of prenatal care have been reduced to the level of pseudoscience. Rather than decry its ineffectiveness, the few critics of American prenatal care that do exist bewail its lack of availability. Current policies have unfortunately had the effect of isolating prenatal care from other equally important aspects of women's healthcare.[27] Moreover, government-sanctioned expansion of prenatal care coverage has not improved overall birth outcomes. For example, utilization of early prenatal care increased by 40 percent among African-American mothers during the

1970s. Yet this increase did not result in a reduction in the number of very-low-birthweight babies born to them.[28]

38   The incentive for prenatal care advocacy in this nation has taken on a life of its own. The goal is no longer to ensure that our mothers and babies have the best outcomes possible. Rather, the imperative is to ensure institutional and bureaucratic survival. The result is that quite often, persons other than pregnant women are the real beneficiaries of American prenatal care.

Almost from its inception, prenatal care has been influenced by a variety of economic and political interests. Given the aura of indispensability that prenatal care has achieved in the United States, it's little wonder that this arena is burgeoning with administrative overgrowth and bureaucracy, especially with regards to high-risk pregnancies. Focusing upon Black mothers as a surrogate high-risk group, for example, Jan Gates-Williams of the University of California in San Francisco tracked the development of prenatal programs in Oakland (Alameda County), California, an area with a large African-American population.[29] She found that between 1978 and 1992, no less than seventeen different perinatal organizations were created or disbanded: "An impressive list of organizations and resources, until one realizes these agencies largely engage in a form of professional bureaucratic recycling." She goes on to lament, "The chronology of Oakland's perinatal health advocacy and infant mortality-related projects reveals interagency and intra-agency overlap and stagnation. This overlap is evident in personnel, in stated project agendas and in the accumulation and control of funding for community low birthweight and infant mortality prevention." For Alameda County, this translated into more advisory/advocacy groups and programs targeted to Oakland's high-risk groups. Despite these efforts, Gates-Williams found that little benefit was realized. The flourishing social service system (Oakland's seventh largest employer in 1986) was unable to favorably impact the very persons for which its many programs, advisory committees, advocacy organizations, and prenatal outreach programs were designed to "help." In the face of widespread prenatal service escalations, Alameda County's racial disparity regarding low birthweight and infant death only worsened. Between 1978 and 1988, low birthweight among Black babies rose 26 percent but fell 12 percent among non-Blacks, for example. Over the same period, infant death among Blacks increased 22 percent but fell 26 percent among non-Blacks. According to Gates-Williams, "These developments have produced yet another service niche: . . . Service providers now have state-subsidized forums for keeping up to date with one another and to systematize the advocacy for more perinatal resources. . . . This affinity for networking has produced a relatively stable, if not fairly lucrative, 'perinatal advocacy and service program oligopoly.'" **39**

The Scientific Basis of Prenatal Care

Once upon a time, there lived a man who spent his days walking the streets of his village, blowing a horn which made a loud and annoying noise. After enduring the nuisance for years, the townspeople grew weary and confronted the man, demanding to know why he persisted with his aggravating habit.

"I do it to keep the elephants away," said the hornblower.

"But there are no elephants within 5,000 miles of here," replied the villagers.

"You see!" the hornblower shrieked, "It's working!"

Even if we accept the appealing premise that prevention saves money, it doesn't address whether prenatal care actually prevents prematurity. The widely held assumption that prenatal care is effective for optimizing pregnancy outcome has allowed prenatal care to escape the scrutiny to which all other medical specialties historically have been subjected. Should we give up on prenatal care? No. But as we shall see, we must take it in a direction that's surprisingly different from where most "experts" presume it should go. A clue to the direction that we must take may be gained by studying what hasn't worked.

Evaluating the Evidence

A number of guidelines have been devised for evaluating the effectiveness of therapeutic medical regimens. In order to evaluate the efficacy of prenatal care, Dr. Kevin Fiscella of the University of Rochester School of Medicine suggests the following criteria:[30]

Temporal Relationship. To be considered effective, medical intervention must precede the outcome. While a relationship between prenatal care and good pregnancy outcomes might seem clear-cut, the relationship may instead be spurious. For example, preterm delivery has been related to fewer

40

prenatal visits. But this seemingly obvious relationship ignores the fact that mothers who deliver prematurely have reduced opportunities for further visits. A woman who delivers at thirty weeks gestation, for instance, will miss her prenatal visits at thirty-four, thirty-six, thirty-seven, thirty-eight, thirty-nine, and forty weeks, thereby creating a statistical quirk known as "preterm delivery bias," which infers that fewer prenatal visits cause prematurity when in reality fewer visits are the *result* of prematurity. This phenomenon can be modified somewhat with several statistical techniques.[31] Nevertheless, these techniques have their limitations, and preterm delivery bias continues to create an artificial dose-response relationship in certain types of studies.

Biologic Plausibility. Medical intervention must have a biologically plausible mechanism that explains the effect of intervention. It may be biologically plausible, in our example, that prenatal care improves pregnancy outcome by modulating maternal risk factors. Yet, as Dr. Fiscella properly points out, the magnitude of this effect is limited by the relatively low prevalence of modifiable risk factors and the availability of effective interventions.[32] To take a case in point, while studies of specialized smoking cessation programs have demonstrated success, routine prenatal care has not been shown to change maternal smoking behavior. The biologic plausibility of prenatal care, moreover, is further weakened by its failure to reduce recurrences of low birthweight among mothers who have previously delivered low-birthweight babies.

Consistency of Research Results. An effective medical intervention should yield replicatible, consistent results when studied by different researchers. But Dr. Fiscella notes that large variations in the scope and magnitude of effects exist among the many studies of prenatal care which purport to show improved pregnancy outcomes. In other words, there is sufficient inconsistency regarding the impact of prenatal care to question its utility.

Alternate Explanations. When evaluating the efficacy of a given medical intervention, researchers must design their studies so as to reduce unanticipated influences which may produce misleading results. Most studies of prenatal care are fraught with confounding factors. As such, conclusions reached by these studies must be tempered with the possibility that unforeseen factors may have influenced their results. For example, we know that mothers who receive inadequate prenatal care are at risk for delivering low-birthweight babies. But many risk factors for low birthweight such as

African-American race
low income
unemployment
low education level
unmarried
unwanted pregnancy
smoking
substance abuse
alcohol abuse
genitourinary infections
domestic violence
psychosocial stress

are also risk factors for inadequate prenatal care, thereby confusing the impact of inadequate prenatal care with antecedent maternal factors that may have contributed to low birthweight.

The idea behind prenatal care is laudable; taking steps to ensure the best possible experience for each mother and child is worthwhile. But much of what we've done over the last forty years hasn't achieved that purpose. According to Dr. David A. Grimes, then with the Centers for Disease Control in Atlanta,

> We Americans have not just accepted new—usually sophisticated—technology uncritically, we have come to worship it. . . . Powerful forces fuel this inexorable drive toward adoption of more and more high technology. One is the fundamental error in most American medicine of rewarding physicians for doing things to patients and not for keeping them well. . . . Most of what we do . . . lacks a firm foundation in science. . . . Dogmas have remained unchallenged because of the widespread confusion between hypothesis and knowledge spawned by uncritical thinking in medicine.[33]

In 1990, the Swedish Council on Technology Assessment in Health Care conducted a conference that investigated the scientific basis of prenatal care.[34] Experts from Europe and North America representing relevant research areas, clinical experience, and healthcare administration participated in the conference. The meeting focused on the available scientific evidence regarding routine programs of prenatal care. The participants determined that the scientific basis for many prenatal care routines is unsatisfactory. In fact, during the 1970s, obstetrics was rated the least scientifically based specialty in all of medicine, receiving the ignominious "wooden spoon" award from Archie Cochrane, Director of MRC Epidemiological Research Unit in Britain. (To be fair, he revoked the award in 1987 after noting an increase in the use of improved research techniques.)[35, 36] That same decade, it was also concluded that the recommendations put forth in 90 percent of published obstetric studies were not scientifically justifiable.[37] Ian Chalmers, Director of the National Perinatal Epidemiology Unit at the Radcliffe Infirmary in Oxford, England, concurs: "Many of the judgments about the value and safety of existing forms of obstetric care continue to be based on evidence that is likely to be invalid."[38]

Back in the United States, Dr. Kevin Fiscella set out to prove the usefulness of prenatal care to himself. But after poring over nearly thirty years of published research papers on the topic, Dr. Fiscella was forced to conclude that: "Current evidence does not satisfy the criteria necessary to establish that prenatal care definitely improves birth outcomes." On the other hand, two previous reviews concluded that prenatal care does improve pregnancy outcomes.[39, 40] However, subsequent publications by some co-authors of those earlier reviews reached conclusions more in keeping with those of Dr. Fiscella.

The work of Dr. Arlene Fink at the University of California in Los Angeles concurs with Fiscella.[41] After evaluating twenty-two published reports on prenatal care, only seven were deemed by Dr. Fink to be of sufficient scientific quality to merit closer assessment: only three of these showed any significant improvements attributable to prenatal care. Over thirty-five years ago, Dr. Sydney H. Kane also questioned its benefits: After examining medical data gathered from over 300,000 deliveries, Dr. Kane found no overall relationship between the number of prenatal visits a mother received and the outcome of her pregnancy.[42] Even when he focused on women who had previously experienced pregnancy losses (in other words, those supposedly most in need of obstetric care), more frequent visits to their obstetricians during subsequent pregnancies did not reduce the chances for recurring tragedy. Dr. Kane's work provides strong evidence that we must be more contrite regarding our ability to appreciably alter the outcomes of many pregnancies.

More recently, Dr. Tina Raine at the University of Washington found that providing ample, adequate prenatal care to a special group of "high-risk" mothers who had previously delivered low-birthweight babies provided no protection whatsoever against repeat performances.[43] The unremitting prematurity rate among American mothers has prompted some to speculate that there's little we can do to appreciably modulate the problem. For example, after studying the issue of prematurity at the University of Chicago, Dr. Robert Mittendorf concluded that America's low-birthweight rate could not **43** be reduced any more than 9 percent below current rates.[44] Dr. J. Martin Tucker at the University of Alabama was only somewhat more optimistic: Based on his own study of Alabama mothers, Dr. Tucker determined that only 23 percent of preterm births were even theoretically avoidable.[45]

Bells and Whistles

Make haste and use all new remedies before they lose their effectiveness.
—Sir William Gall

Our nation's medical culture is rife with the attitude that if something can be done, it must be done no matter how ineffective or unproven it may be.[46] In obstetrics, no stone can be left unturned, irrespective of the relevance or usefulness of the regimen being prescribed. Accordingly, mothers expect that when they pose a problem to their doctors, something will be done about it; whether the treatment actually makes a difference is entirely secondary to the appearance that steps are being taken.

In this nation, action is always favored over conservative management— even when watchful waiting is the most appropriate course. Adherence to this philosophy brought American mothers the diethylstilbestrol (DES) fiasco thirty years ago: Frustrated by their inability to prevent miscarriages, American obstetricians seized upon DES when it was suggested that this synthetic hormone could arrest the problem.[47] It was only years later that we learned of its horrible long-term side effects: infertility, reproductive tract malformations and malignancies began to appear in young girls and women exposed to DES in utero. Many died.

Most obstetricians aren't scientists, they're clinicians: easy prey for hortatory medical hucksters. Makers of obstetric-related drugs and devices exploit these circumstances, sending armies of salesmen into the offices of American obstetricians on missions of persuasion. Much of what many doctors learn about "advancements" in the field comes not from objective medical journals or unbiased symposiums but from the lips of company representatives intent on selling a product. The Hippocratic Oath that each new physician must take entreats them to "do no harm." But when we prescribe unproven or worthless regimens to our mothers, we do them economic harm. In an environment where unfounded and expensive treatments divert money away from rudimentary but fundamentally sound practices, women—especially poor ones—are harmed because their needs are obscured by the bells and whistles of deluxe prenatal care. If the available treatment options are costly and ineffective (or unproven), there should be no imperative to offer them. Unfortunately, this option is usually not even considered. To deny a mother treatment, however worthless the treatment may be, is to deny her nevertheless—something we can't seem to do as long as she's able to afford it.

Exhibit A: Cervical Cerclage

An example of our romance with unproven obstetric treatments harkens back to the early part of this century when a surgical technique was introduced whereby the mother's cervix was literally sewn shut in the hope of preventing preterm delivery. Clinical trials were conducted on the cerclage procedure between the 1950s and the 1980s, but none were randomized clinical trials (i.e., the most reliable type of clinical research). Most simply compared pregnancy outcomes in women after they received cerclage with the outcomes of their pregnancies before the procedure, a completely inadequate basis for inferring effectiveness. Interestingly, the fetal survival rate of these 15 studies (63 percent to 89 percent) is surprisingly similar to the 70- to 85-percent likelihood of survival cited by L. S. Bakketeig for women with previously curtailed pregnancies for whom no special measures were taken during subsequent gestations.[48]

To make matters worse, when randomized clinical studies were finally done, they disclosed that not only did the procedure not improve pregnancy outcomes, but women who underwent the surgery experienced more frequent occurrences of other pregnancy complications.[49-51] Prompted by the data, one cerclage researcher stated that "So far, no experimentally derived evidence is available to justify such practice."[52] Nevertheless, many obstetricians still consider the benefits of cerclage to be unequivocal. This philosophy has led to very frequent use of the procedure around the world, reaching a cerclage rate of 18 percent at one maternity hospital during the 1970s—an astounding figure given that the underlying problem for which the cerclage procedure was invented only occurs in about 1 percent of pregnant women.[53] As one weary cerclage researcher sagely notes, "Once again, we may find that firmly held clinical convictions do not stand the test of scientific scrutiny."[54]

Exhibit B: Tocolytic Drugs

Tocolytic drugs are another example of an obstetric treatment detached from **45** supporting scientific data. Tocolytics are supposed to exert their effect by causing the contracting uterus to relax, thereby retarding the prematurity process. Unfortunately, the evidence that these drugs, when administered orally for long-term therapy, actually prolong pregnancy is unconvincing. Nevertheless, the use of these compounds has become accepted standard practice in many parts of the United States. The failure of these drugs is no secret. As one popular obstetrics textbook advises obstetricians-in-training: "It has become almost obligatory to begin general discussions of tocolytic drugs by pointing out that preterm birth rates have remained stable despite the use of millions of tablets and ampules of these powerful medications."[55]

Over 15 years ago, Dr. Marc J. N. C. Keirse concluded that the most widely used type of oral tocolytic drugs was of no value when it came to prolonging the pregnancies of women with preterm labor, yet the use of these drugs is as popular as ever.[56] More recently, Dr. George A. Macones at Jefferson Medical College in Philadelphia reached similar conclusions after carefully reviewing published medical reports regarding the effectiveness of the long-term use of these medications.[57] Among the research trials on this topic, the recurring theme is one of ineffectiveness and undue risk, raising the question as to why this medical regimen has become so widespread. Indeed, Dr. Macones makes a plea to his obstetric colleagues around the country regarding the results of his research: "We realize this finding is in direct contrast to physician practices at many centers. . . . We would encourage all physicians to weigh carefully the potential risks and benefits of therapy for each patient before embarking on long-term oral . . . therapy."

More recently, the industry has developed an "improved" way to administer these drugs to mothers: by slowly, continuously pumping them under the skin. Naturally, the necessary equipment is expensive. Less obvious are the benefits that accrue. Two randomized clinical trials found no benefits from the subcutaneous pump device.[58, 59] After evaluating this new technology, Dr. Jeffery G. Bailey at Ohio State University concluded that the expense and the lack of supporting data should "discourage recommendations of its general clinical use." Both the American College of Obstetricians and Gynecologists and the Food and Drug Administration agree.[60, 61] Nevertheless, this new device has not been confined to the clinical laboratory until its benefit can be proven. Rather, obstetricians have embraced this new treatment and its high cost without evidence that it's a remarkably better treatment modality. Many swear by these drugs, confidently asserting that their use spells the difference between prematurity and a full-term delivery. What they are unwilling to address is the fact that mothers are just as likely to achieve full-term gestations without these compounds.

46

Exhibit C: The HUAM Scam

The latest and perhaps most disturbing display of our prenatal system's penchant for ever more technology is the home uterine activity monitoring (HUAM) device. Although the effectiveness of HUAM is unsettled, the cost of this new device—roughly sixty to eighty dollars daily per patient—would suggest that its utility is clear-cut.[62] It isn't.

A feature of HUAM that would imply its usefulness stems from the ability of the device to detect uterine contractions that the mother herself cannot perceive, providing an "early warning system" for preterm labor. But despite its theoretic utility, the actual effectiveness of HUAM has been questioned by many from its inception. Dr. David A. Grimes, a nationally recognized researcher at the University of California in San Francisco and a vocal critic of HUAM research, has lamented for years the introduction of this new device before adequate, credible research had accumulated.[63] In 1992, Dr. Grimes concluded that, "The existing studies suffer from many serious if not fatal methodologic flaws. . . . Trials of home uterine activity . . . have not met accepted standards of scientific rigor. . . . Until the efficacy of home uterine activity monitoring has been established, this procedure should not be used clinically."

In the largest, most extensive assessment of HUAM to date, Dr. Lawrence DeVoe at the Medical College of Georgia found that the device did not confer additional benefit beyond that provided by intensive, conscientious care.[64] Both the American College of Obstetricians and Gynecologists and the U.S. Preventive Services Task Force have refused to endorse "this expensive and burdensome system."[65, 66] Indeed, on the eve of the American College of Obstetricians and Gynecologists' preparations to re-examine the subject of HUAM, the two major HUAM companies (which have since merged) attempted to distract the College from the facts by encouraging obstetricians to mount a letter-writing campaign urging official endorsement of HUAM. Form letters spelling out the companies' party line were conveniently mailed to every obstetrician in America (all that was required was their signature and a stamp) in the hopes that the College would legitimize what objective research has been unable to do.

The advent and dissemination of HUAM technology in the face of un-proven utility is a case study of how American prenatal care providers embrace ever higher levels of sophistication and expense without producing **47** concomitant improvements in overall pregnancy outcomes. Widespread clinical acceptance of HUAM has occurred far in advance of any consistent, convincing evidence that it's a genuinely effective treatment modality. Meanwhile, the HUAM industry thrives on the yet-to-be-proven assertion that their product actually reduces the risk of prematurity. But home uterine activity monitoring has achieved such a following among some obstetricians that those who fail to offer HUAM as an available treatment option arguably fall below the "standard of care," thereby evoking the potential medicolegal risks that such behavior poses. Thus, HUAM—while awaiting the accumulation of sufficient scientific evidence that it actually works—has skyrocketed from a plausible idea to a quasi-necessity over the course of a single decade. The comments of Dr. Robert L. Goldenberg at the University of Alabama provide insight into why this has occurred:

> The finances at stake are tremendous. Commercial companies charge in the range of 80 dollars per day per patient for the use of this technology. One can make various assumptions about its potential use, but if somewhere between 10 and 20 percent of the four million women in the United States having babies each year are classified as high risk for preterm delivery, and monitoring is used an average of 8 or 10 weeks during each pregnancy, the potential income to be derived from its use is the range of two to four billion dollars a year.[67]

Exhibit D: Ultrasound as a Toy

Everybody likes ultrasound—especially expectant mothers. But obstetric ul-trasonography is frequently performed at the whim of obstetricians for no particular reason. In an increasingly competitive business, it's often used as a marketing tool, for entertainment, or for such nondescript reasons as promoting maternal "bonding" with the fetus. Meanwhile, the cost of an in-office ultrasound machine is passed along to patients via direct billing or indirectly with increased prenatal fees.

The utility of obstetric ultrasound depends upon the expertise and skill of the person actually performing the assessment. But as it presently stands, any American obstetrician who wishes to perform ultrasound need only purchase a machine and he/she's in business because there are no

uniform or enforced standards of quality to which they must adhere. Dr. Harris J. Finberg, a nationally renowned radiologist who's devoted his ca-
48 reer to obstetric ultrasound, concluded from data gleaned from a study of American obstetric ultrasound that: "Obstetrical ultrasound, as it is currently being practiced in the United States, may fall below the standards of quality now achieved in Europe."[68] Others have also hypothesized that European ultrasound screening programs—conducted in obstetric sonography centers where scanning conforms to a uniform protocol—are superior to those in America. Dr. Finberg's concerns are echoed by Dr. James P. Crane of Washington University in St. Louis: "More rigorous training of individuals who perform and interpret obstetric ultrasonographic examinations is appropriate."[69] The widespread availability of ultrasound technology to any American obstetrician who can afford a machine shows how technology tends to migrate away from those with proper training and experience to those who simply want to capture market share of a lucrative technique. With the recent introduction of so-called "three-dimensional" ultrasound, the entertainment value of ultrasound is at a premium, even though many are uncertain how much extra diagnostic utility this expensive new treatment modality will produce.

Inappropriate or unnecessary use of an attractive technique like ultrasound adds to mounting prenatal costs and may occasionally lead to improper diagnoses. The seductive nature of this modality is apparent—one ultrasound examination invariably seems to make another necessary. Additionally, Dr. Manuel Porto of the University of California in Irvine notes that malpractice suits for missed fetal anomaly detection on routine obstetric ultrasound examinations appear to be increasing;[70] and anomalies are more likely to be missed when routine second-trimester ultrasound evaluations are done in obstetricians' offices.

For better or worse, ultrasound assessment has become a mainstay of American prenatal care. Therefore, it's incumbent upon mothers to ensure that they're not worse off for having undergone one. It's always appropriate to ask your doctor about his/her ultrasound training. How much specific, supervised instruction did he/she receive? Generally, newer OB/GYN's receive at least some training in the technique during their residencies, but few are sufficiently expert at ultrasound to be considered "centers of excellence." Ask your doctor about any special certification he/she may have in obstetric ultrasound. Unless he/she has received "fellowship" training (two to three years of additional training after his/her residency) and/or AIUM (the American Institute of Ultrasound in Medicine) certification, you may not be receiving the level of diagnostic acumen that you think you are. Before consenting to an ultrasound, find out if there are other facilities in your area with a higher level of expertise and/or certification. Frequently there will be, especially if you live in a metropolitan area. Obviously, because ultrasound has become an economic and prestige issue for many obstetricians, they may not automatically offer you options, especially when it comes to an initial screening ultrasound.

Exhibit E: Vitamins et Cetera

Prenatal vitamins are the time-honored, prototypical medication given to expectant mothers. Purportedly to augment the nutritional well-being of pregnant women in the United States, prenatal vitamin and iron supplementation has become so commonplace that, according to Dr. David A. Nagey at the University of Maryland, it's become "almost a symbol of prenatal care."[71] Unfortunately, seventeen medical studies of prenatal vitamin supplementation have not demonstrated any benefit from this traditional intervention.[72] Although this lapse is harmless, many obstetricians are even less informed regarding medications that mothers with certain conditions actually do need during pregnancy. According to Dr. Roy M. Pitkin at the University of California in Los Angeles, mothers with serious conditions are sometimes denied medication because of the mistaken belief that they're harmful to the fetus.[73] While some drugs are best avoided during gestation, there are times when the benefits of certain medications outweigh any potential risks. In many cases Dr. Pitkin thinks concerns about fetal risks are shortsighted: "It's in a fetus' best interest to have a healthy mother." In support of Pitkin's concerns, a survey of Washington, D.C., obstetricians found that fully one-third would advise mothers who took a common epilepsy medication to abort their pregnancies despite the fact that the drug increases the risk of certain birth defects by only 1 to 2 percent.[74]

Guided by the principle of "helping" mothers but unencumbered by any real need to demonstrate their effectiveness, worthless nostrums such as prenatal vitamins are passing as standard care while genuinely useful treatments are ignored or avoided. A particularly tragic example of an effective treatment which has been ignored is a group of medications known as corticosteroids: as long ago as 1981, seven well-executed research trials demonstrated that corticosteroid administration significantly improved the outcomes of premature babies. By 1990, the number of studies had risen to twelve—over 3,000 mothers had been evaluated.[75] Despite excellent scientific support for the use of corticosteroid drugs, the National Institute of Health noted in 1994 that only 12 to 18 percent of mothers delivering babies weighing less than 1,500 grams were receiving this clearly beneficial treatment.[76] As Dr. David Grimes laments, "Because of this delay in adopting useful therapy, tens of thousands of neonates died needlessly in the interim, and our nation squandered millions of healthcare dollars treating preventable complications of prematurity."[77] A study by Dr. William J. Hueston of the University of Wisconsin illustrates the incongruity. Dr. Hueston found that women presenting with preterm uterine contractions but no evidence of actual preterm labor were frequently overtreated with agents of "equivocal benefit" (i.e., many types of tocolytics) between 1995 and 1997.[78] At the same time, only one in three of those with genuine preterm labor received corticosteroids.

Future Mischief

A new test which supposedly differentiates those at high risk for preterm delivery from those at low risk was recently approved by the Food and Drug Administration. Known as the fetal fibronectin (FFN) assay, this simple test has shown promise in preliminary studies.[79, 80] Among symptomatic mothers with negative FFN tests, over 98 percent will avoid prematurity over the ensuing one to two weeks. Although only a minority of those with positive screens will go on to have preterm deliveries, the reassurance that a negative FFN assay can provide is invaluable, allowing mothers to avoid unnecessary, expensive prenatal mischief.

As is any promising new diagnostic tool, FFN screening is ripe for misuse. Indeed, some practitioners now perform routine FFN screens every few weeks on patients deemed to be at high risk for preterm labor. Because the test's prognostic power has been oversold to patients, however, some have become fairly dependent on the test even when there is no indication for its administration. Ultimately, the results of any screening test performed on the wrong patients at the wrong time for the wrong reasons are bound to be misleading. To illustrate, Dr. Ayala Revah of the University of Toronto reviewed twenty-four prospective, blinded trials of FFN screening.[81] In those studies where the screen was performed on the proper patients (i.e., those with significant signs and symptoms of preterm labor), a negative test result was quite predictive: only two percent of patients delivered within seven to ten days of the test. But the reliability of the screen diminished considerably when it was performed without an indication on symptom-free women. In fact, among asymptomatic women with positive FFN screens, only 43 per- **51** cent actually delivered prior to thirty-four weeks and only 28 percent delivered prior to thirty-seven weeks. Moreover, over 40 percent of those delivering within seven to twenty-eight days of the screening test had negative test results. Dr. Revah advises against the use of FFN screening for symptomless patients, in part to avoid "unnecessary or harmful interventions." On the other hand, Revah also warns that a negative test result in this situation may be falsely reassuring. Unfortunately, a new standard of care is slowly evolving which includes routine FFN screening—a standard based on patient demand, misunderstanding of the role of FFN screening, and the encouragement of medical one-upmanship. As with other misbegotten standards of prenatal care, the burden of proof will shift from those who adhere to the new standard and onto those who sought to prevent its widespread assimilation.

An obstetrician's desire to offer a remedy—and the medical industry's eagerness to supply it—are not sufficient grounds to permit the widespread dissemination of worthless or inappropriate regimens. A mother's willingness to endure an unproven therapy in the name of helping her baby does not render the treatment more effective. Worse, it sets a dangerous precedent whereby others will use her experience as justification to try the treatment on others. In such scenarios, individual testimonials supplant hard numbers. Over time, procedures such as cerclage gain credibility through the accumulation of anecdote.

What We Can Do about It: Step Two

Technology Must Be Reigned In

We must stop falling into the trap of "newer" or "different" when it comes to prenatal care. Our nation's awful maternity status doesn't justify the rush to well-intended but ineffective care. With each obstetrical wild goose chase that diverts our attention, we stray further from genuinely useful, though less flashy, strategies for helping our mothers and their babies. The ongoing incursion of unproven, insufficiently evaluated "breakthroughs" has done little for prenatal care except increase its expense. All future obstetric innovations must be subjected to ample, rigorous medical research (indeed,

52

firmly entrenched obstetric rituals should also be scrutinized). Before subjecting American mothers to any further "improvements" in prenatal care, scientific evidence should be evaluated by expert obstetric review panels convened to determine the sufficiency, appropriateness, and methodologic rigor of supporting medical research. New diagnostic and therapeutic modalities must have convincing, reproducible supporting evidence gleaned from unbiased, objective researchers before manufacturers are allowed to reap the profits that such advancements produce. New prenatal technology must never again be allowed to become the standard of care until its utility is shown to be clear-cut. Guidelines for utilization of prenatal technology must be established and strictly followed.

The tendency of new technologies to expand beyond the arena of their original intent reduces their utility and increases costs as they are put to inappropriate uses. Novel uses of established technologies may sometimes produce genuine benefit—other times they create needless intervention. Excursions of technology beyond its original intent must be controlled. When permitted, they must proceed under close scrutiny with well-designed research protocols so as to maximize efficacy and safety. At the same time, we must be realistic. Instead of more research, perhaps we should settle for better research. As Peter Huber advised: "It is perhaps comforting to declare that we need more research. But that statement is always trite and often wrong. Worse still, calls for more research provide great comfort to junk scientists who will find there subtle support for their own idiosyncratic crusades."[82]

Many "advancements" are the product of optimistic but sometimes incomplete medical research. As more data is accumulated through subsequent studies, a clearer understanding is frequently achieved. More is learned about how a treatment works. Over time, more realistic expectations are gained—subsequent pronouncements regarding the effectiveness of a given "breakthrough" are usually less optimistic than were the initial claims. In most cases, the advancement is downgraded from "miracle cure" to "useful tool." Then, somewhere along the line, reports crop up regarding misuse or unforeseen side effects.

A prime example regarding the natural history of a wonder drug may be found in the story of cortisone, a well-known medicine now in widespread use. When "compound E," as it was originally called, was first used decades ago, the results it produced were hailed as nothing short of a miracle, and its discoverers were even awarded the Nobel Prize. One bedridden patient regained his ability to walk after a short course of this drug. But in time, it became apparent that compound E was not without its problems. With prolonged use, higher and higher doses became necessary to produce the desired clinical response. Chronic use of this drug also resulted **53** in a host of unexpected problems including diabetes, Cushing's disease, osteoporosis, and more. In a relatively brief span of time, cortisone had fallen from grace. Only with sufficient research and clinical experience did cortisone find its proper place in certain medical regimens. Indeed, when prudently administered and monitored, cortisone can produce dramatic, even lifesaving results.

Similar experiences have befallen other one-time medical marvels: birth-control pills, intrauterine contraceptive devices, and even antibiotics have cycled through the panacea-to-pariah-to-prudent-use circuit. Others, such as thalidomide, DES, and "Phen-Fen" fared less well. The point is that less is known about newer treatment regimens—frequently, the "big picture" becomes evident only after years of use. In some cases, a price is paid by patients who clamor onto a new regimen only to find that the innovation is ultimately found to be worthless—or worse, harmful to them or their babies. Do not fall prey to the fanfare of a product or regimen that's "newer" or "different" than more well-studied therapeutic modalities unless your prenatal care provider can convince you—not with anecdotes or testimonials—of its superiority as described below.

There are different types of medical research, but the most credible is the randomized clinical trial, or RCT. Generally, data generated from this type of research is the most valuable but also the most scarce because RCT's are the most difficult type of clinical research to conduct. Treatments shown to be effective via lesser research techniques are often found to be worthless when scrutinized by prospective RCT's. Don't be swayed by inferior research reports. Obviously, most parents lack the scientific background to discern good clinical research from less important or frankly bad studies. Some resources which may be useful when it comes to studying a given obstetric topic include:

- *The Cochrane Database.* This electronic database is revised quarterly, thereby providing regular updates of medical/obstetrical research from around the world. Subscriptions may be purchased through the American College of Physicians (www.acponline.org).
- *Medline.* Access to Medline, an online catalogue of published research which is regularly updated, is easiest through medical libraries located in most metropolitan hospitals and medical centers.

- *Index Medicus.* Available in text or electronic formats, Index Medicus is a catalogue of all published medical research. It may be found at most metropolitan medical libraries and is updated monthly. This publication only gives the name of the study, names of the authors and the journal in which it appears; it does not provide any text from the study, so you'll have to do some digging.

- *The American College of Obstetricians and Gynecologists (ACOG).* ACOG publishes a "Technical Bulletin" and an "Educational Bulletin" which summarize ACOG's opinions on a variety of obstetric issues. Many of the more recent and more relevant studies are cited in the Bulletins. The Bulletins aren't updated as frequently as other sources and the opinions rendered are usually "middle of the road" and unprovocative, as one might expect literature published by governing bodies would be. However, they may provide a useful starting point for one's review of the literature on a given obstetric topic and may be obtained by writing to:

  The American College of Obstetricians and Gynecologists
  409 12th Street, SW
  P.O. Box 96920
  Washington, D.C. 20090–6920

- *Effective Care in Pregnancy and Childbirth,* Volume 2 (I. Chalmers, M. Enkin, M. J. N. C. Keirse, editors, Oxford: Oxford University Press, 1989). A nice resource to have regarding obstetric issues. Because it's in print form, it necessarily lags behind other media from a "cutting-edge" perspective. But it's also a good starting point for researching a particular obstetric topic. Its electronic cousin (The Cochrane Database) compliments this text nicely.

When scanning the obstetric literature, remember RCT's trump all other types of clinical research. But be careful, even some RCT's are poorly executed, reaching invalid or incorrect conclusions. To complicate matters further, some medical researchers accept funding or other material support/remuneration from medical manufacturers to conduct studies—even RCT's—on their medical products, thereby raising questions as to how truly objective research can be when it has essentially been purchased by the manufacturers. Which type of medical research would you find more credible—studies funded by a manufacturer with a vested interest in the outcome (e.g., those companies which sell home uterine activity monitoring devices, sub-cutaneous tocolytic pumps, etc.) or studies conducted by independent, objective researchers? Upon which type of research would you want your care-giver to base his/her clinical decisions? Thus, it is important to know if a given study was funded by a private medical manufacturer; this fact will generally be acknowledged somewhere in the text of studies published in reputable journals.

Therapeutic regimens whose efficacy is largely supported by non-RCT research should be suspect. (Of note, a review of scientific articles published in a major American obstetrics journal during 1996 revealed that only 11 percent of the studies were RCT's.)[83] RCT's of a given regimen which reach contradictory conclusions should also raise a red flag about the utility of the regimen. Clues that the study being reviewed is an RCT may be found by certain key words in the title or text of the study:

- *prospective*
- *randomized*
- *double-blinded*

Clues that the study isn't an RCT are suggested by the absence of the above key words and/or the presence of other ones:

- *retrospective*
- *non-randomized*
- *case report*
- *case-controlled study*
- *cohort study*

Medicine is a competitive business, albeit not yet to the point where doctors are handing out toasters. Nevertheless, a subtle game of medical one-upmanship exists among practitioners. As a result, the interval between the debut and the widespread acceptance of a new tool/technique is relatively short. If Mrs. Smith's obstetrician is using the latest technology, her neighbor's obstetrician will soon be using it too as patients and doctors alike ride the wave of innovation. But a product's speed of assimilation isn't necessarily a reflection of its effectiveness.

Lost in the shuffle is the fact that few obstetric "breakthroughs" actually result in significantly better outcomes for the mothers who use them.

At best, many new products are merely "as good as" standard obstetric fare. Dollar for dollar, however, newer products are sometimes less effec-
56   tive than cheaper, older, less-racy therapeutic iterations (i.e., they're less "cost-effective"). Moreover, better-established regimens are also more likely to be covered by a given health insurer. An insurer's unwillingness to cover a new regimen could be a reflection of many possibilities, some of which may have little to do with mothers' well-being (see chapter 4).

On the other hand, better pregnancy outcomes ultimately save insurance companies money. The hesitancy of some carriers to pay for a device like the home uterine activity monitor suggests that some in the insurance industry have a different interpretation of the published medical data about home monitoring than does the home monitoring industry itself. Therefore, it behooves the patient to understand why a particular course of action is being pursued by her prenatal caregiver.

Just because a new technique is available, it doesn't mean that a given prenatal care provider has expertise with it. There are virtually no requirements a doctor must fulfill before using or administering many new tools or techniques. In some cases, a doctor will provide a new diagnostic or therapeutic tool for his patients after attending a weekend seminar or seven-day course (often provided by the company which sells the new tool). This is not always sufficient time to master a new technique. In other cases, the doctor is only required to prescribe a new obstetric modality; thereafter, a service company takes over. An example of this arrangement is the terbutaline pump, mentioned earlier. After the obstetrician orders the device for a given mother, the service company teaches the mother how to use the device and determines her dose of medication. Except for signing orders which are mailed to him after the system is up and running, the doctor is largely out of the loop. As a result, the doctor needn't have any understanding of the terbutaline pump regimen or the scanty scientific evidence that supports its use. Therefore, it's important to query your doctor regarding his/her personal training, clinical experience, and scientific understanding of this or any new tools. Better yet, ask your caregiver for reading material on the topic. A well-read doctor should have no trouble providing or guiding you to the literature which convinced him/her a given treatment modality was right for you. Beware of literature published or provided by the new product's manufacturer; it's rarely unbiased. Beware of caregivers who cannot provide objective medical literature: it may not exist or your caregiver may not have read it, leading to inevitable questions as to why you should be following a given regimen or using a particular device.

Questions for the Obstetrician

To avoid being swept up in the rush towards technology and new regimens, there are certain essential questions that a mother should ask her prenatal care provider:

- How long has a given "innovation" been around?
- What is the evidence that a given regimen/device actually works?
- Are there other, more traditional treatments that are equally effective?
- Why do you believe that this particular regimen is right for me?
- Does this particular technique require special training or expertise? Do you have it? Is there someone who does?

A prime example (again) is obstetric ultrasound. This useful but expensive technology has a variety of features that encourage misuse during gestation:

- Ultrasound appears to be safe for use during pregnancy. The rudiments of obstetric ultrasound are easy to learn.
- Ultrasound is very popular among mothers.
- In-office ultrasound may be used as a clinical "centerpiece" to attract or keep patients.

3. Money

In Every Town, a Temple

In contrast to this country's lowly status in regard to low-birthweight deliveries, our skill at treating premature infants is the best in the world—caring for more than 400,000 low-birthweight babies each year has provided ample practice. No other field salvages more life per patient than neonatology. While other medical specialties may prolong the lives of sick patients by months or years, the span of life that neonatologists frequently preserve is measured in decades. The neonatal intensive care unit (NICU) is a showcase of genuine medical progress. But to the same extent that America's overabundance of obstetricians has done little to reduce prematurity, the mounting number of NICU's has worsened rather than helped the problem.

When it comes to highly complex intensive care, quantity and quality go hand in hand. Consequently, patient outcomes tend to be better at busy, well-practiced facilities. Indeed, an inverse relationship exists between the number of selected procedures performed at a given medical center and post-procedure mortality. Facilities that perform more of a given procedure such as cardiac bypass or hip replacement surgery have lower mortality rates. To illustrate this practice effect, Dr. James G. Jollis at Duke University examined the relationship between the number of percutaneous transluminal coronary angioplasty (PTCA) procedures performed and associated complications.[1] Dr. Jollis examined the outcomes of roughly 218,000 patients from 1987 through 1990. The in-hospital mortality among patients undergoing PTCA ranged from 2.5 percent among the busiest hospitals to 3.9 percent among those with the lowest patient volume. The need for cardiac bypass surgery after PTCA also increased from 2.8 percent at the busiest centers to 5.3 percent at the least busy facilities. Unfortunately, the "practice makes perfect" philosophy at the heart of a successful, time-tested system of neonatal care is being undermined.

A Short Course in Regionalization

In the early 1970s, a nationwide effort to improve obstetric and neonatal **59** (i.e., "perinatal") care was initiated with the goal of establishing regional hospitals for acutely complicated pregnancies. Regionalization of extremely expensive commodities like NICU's permitted excellent care for premature or sick newborns in a fashion that was more affordable than the alternative of placing NICU's in every hospital across the country. There are three different levels of perinatal hospital care. While specifics will vary from state to state, the criteria listed by Susan L. Powell of the University of Washington provides some general guidelines:[2]

Level I
- Licensed obstetric unit.
- < 500 births per year or absence of one or more of the optional level II criteria.

Level II
- ≥ 500 births per year.
- Board-certified OB/GYN's and pediatricians on staff.
- Laboratory technicians and anesthesiologists available at all times.
- Ultrasound available in the hospital.
- Maximum nurse-patient ratio of 1:4 for newborn intermediate care.

Level III–Level II criteria plus:
- Neonatal intensive care unit (NICU) able to provide full life-support, resuscitation, and monitoring services for newborns.
- Staff with post-residency training in perinatology, neonatology and obstetric, neonatal and pediatric anesthesia.
- Staff OB/GYN's specializing in ultrasound, amniocentesis, and endocrinology/infertility.
- Staff pediatricians specializing in neurology, hematology, genetics, and cardiology.
- Maximum registered nurse-patient ratio of 1:2 for NICU patients.
- Regular experience with severe respiratory distress requiring mechanical ventilation and with congenital cardiac disease.
- Intensive care unit for high-risk maternity patients pre- and post-delivery.
- CAT (computerized axial tomography) scanner available in the hospital.

• Established program for accepting and directing maternal and neonatal transports.

(Reprinted with permission of Mosby, Inc., from S. L. Powell, V. L. Holt, D. E. Hickok, T. Easterling, F. A. Connell. "Recent Changes in Delivery Site of Low-Birthweight Infants in Washington: Impact on Birth Weight–Specific Morality." *American Journal of Obstetrics and Gynecology.* 173(1995)1585.)

By concentrating patients from one area into a single "level III" center, obstetric and NICU personnel were assured of having sufficient experience to maintain their skills so as to give each baby the best possible care. For preterm newborns, these centers offer many benefits including immediate access to a plethora of specialized services critical to the care of extremely fragile babies. In some cases, regionalization represents the difference between life and death.

We've known for decades that lower mortality rates of low-birthweight infants accompany more intensive care: L. S. Bakketeig noted in Norway during the 1960s and '70s that first-week mortality rates were highest where access to intensive perinatal care was lowest.[3] Likewise, in the late 1970s, Dr. Nigel Paneth at Columbia University examined mortality rates of neonates weighing from 500 to 2,250 grams in New York City.[4] Among 13,560 low-birthweight babies, the adjusted neonatal death rate was significantly different for each of the three levels of care: 16 percent at level I centers, 17 percent at level II centers and 13 percent at level III centers. Dr. Paneth's data indicated that the risk of death for low-birthweight babies increased 1.3-fold at "outpost" (i.e., level I or II) hospitals. Dr. Paneth concluded that, "The data suggests that some of the excess mortality in level II units might be avoided if these units made more extensive use of the transfer system to refer infants promptly for level III care. . . . To attain the maximum effect, it seems necessary also to ensure that as many low-birthweight infants as possible are delivered in level III hospitals."

Most recently, Susan L. Powell at the University of Washington conducted an eleven-year review of low-birthweight infants to evaluate the effects of perinatal regionalization.[5] Powell's retrospective study of newborns weighing 500 to 2,499 grams between 1980 and 1991 found that the percentage of low-birthweight babies born at level III centers rose from 1980 to 1988, suggesting that regionalization was being practiced in Washington. This phenomenon was confirmed by the research of Dr. Roger A. Rosenblatt, also at the University of Washington School of Medicine.[6] In both cases, regionalization was associated with better survival rates of low-birth-weight babies delivered at level III centers when compared to outpost hospitals. However, Powell's report noted a trend away from regionalization in Washington after 1988 and concluded that some of the deaths of low-birth-weight babies born at outpost hospitals as a result of deregionalization could have been prevented by prenatal referral to level III centers.

The very high mortality rate that occurs during the first few hours of life at outpost hospitals underscores the benefit of delivery at a level III center over neonatal transport to a level III center. Even if excellent transport is available in rural areas, the delay involved places very low birthweight infants at risk. Dr. Lula O. Lubchenco at the University of Colorado evaluated the effect of prenatal versus neonatal transport of babies weighing 500 to 1,499 grams.[7] One group of infants was delivered at a level III perinatal center; the other group consisted of infants delivered at five level I hospitals, then transported to a level III center. During the four-year study, 174 very-low-birth-weight babies delivered at the level III center while 297 delivered at outpost hospitals. At the level III facility, there was a significant reduction in fetal deaths and neonatal complications. Dr. Lubchenco concluded that for the smallest babies, care at level III centers may improve outcomes. To confirm this phenomenon, Dr. Ronald J. Ozminkowski at the University of Michigan analyzed a series of nineteen studies which addressed the issue.[8] Like Dr. Lubchenco, Ozminkowski found that the overall odds of death for newborns weighing 2,500 grams or less who were delivered at level III institutions were considerably lower than those born at outpost hospitals and then transferred. His data suggests that neonatal mortality may be reduced "by avoiding risks related to transfer of newborns to the NICU and by more timely and efficacious diagnosis and treatment of mothers and infants by more qualified staff with better resources." According to Dr. William Kitchen of the University of Melbourne, "The much lower prevalence of serious handicaps found in survivors born in tertiary (level III) centers compared with those transferred postnatally is of considerable clinical significance to infants, their families and the community; it justifies the inconvenience and family stresses that transfer in utero to a tertiary center may impose."[9]

Increasingly, hospitals in the United States are seeking to develop their own NICU's in regions already served by level III centers. Despite its documented success, entrepreneurial forces have placed perinatal regionalization in jeopardy.[10-15] In an increasingly competitive market, many hospitals have expanded their facilities in hopes of achieving greater market share. This is especially true of perinatal services because they tend to generate relatively larger hospital revenues than do other hospital-based medical specialties. As a result, some better-equipped level II centers are providing perinatal services to high-risk patients that they previously would have referred to level III institutions. The philosophy of regionalization is increasingly being eroded by economic rather than medical motivations: Under managed care, healthcare groups may be economically driven to develop their own perinatal programs in order to sell their services to the public, further jeopardizing perinatal regionalization. In many instances, competing hospitals will develop less than full-service (level II) NICU's, equipped to handle all but the smallest and sickest neonates. Other times, physicians will simply elect to keep their patients under their care at outpost hospitals instead of transferring the newborn or pregnant mother to level III centers. Sometimes the decision not to transfer is appropriate. But to the extent that a patient is kept at her local hospital, control over her care and the revenue her care generates will be kept local. It is also more convenient for the patient and her family if she stays at an institution closer to home. As such, physicians and hospital administrators based at hospitals without level III facilities compete for mothers and neonates served by regional centers. In some circumstances, population growth warrants the development of additional level III NICU's. In a rapidly growing metropolitan area, for example, the expanding population provides ample experience and revenues to justify the creation of new perinatal regions. Other times, the creation of a new facility within an established referral region reflects nothing more than a grab for market penetration. The result is needless expenditure for services already available within the region.

While deregionalization of neonatal care offers a boon to the local physician and a convenience to mother and family, the impact upon premature infants is less than reassuring. Ongoing care at an outpost hospital presents the same risk to its patients that under-utilized coronary bypass programs run—insufficient experience. As such, the outcomes of newborns in these units may be inferior to those at larger regional centers. A study mentioned earlier which was conducted by Susan L. Powell at the University of Washington analyzed more than 43,000 low-birthweight neonates between 1980 and 1991 to determine if the place of delivery had an effect on neonatal mortality rates.[16] Among infants weighing less than 2,000 grams, delivery at outpost hospitals correlated with significantly higher mortality rates. Specifically, the neonatal death rate at outpost hospitals increased almost twofold over that noted at level III centers.

Supply and Demand

The law of supply and demand is the driving principle of commerce and free enterprise but not for the healthcare industry in America. For decades, members of the medical profession have exempted themselves from the direct relationship between the supply of service providers and the fees they can demand. Across the twentieth century, as the number of doctors has increased, their incomes have also increased. The only challenge that their burgeoning numbers posed was that of finding enough disease to keep everyone busy. For enterprising physicians, this hasn't been a problem: as the supply of doctors has expanded, the threshold for conditions that require medical supervision has fallen. In other words, doctors have gone looking for business. Indeed, it's interesting how certain types of diseases increase in proportion to the number of specialists available to treat them. In Maine, for example, a dramatic increase in back problems requiring surgery occurred after that state experienced a large influx of neurosurgeons.[17] Did back problems spontaneously burgeon in Maine when the neurosurgeons arrived? No; the glut of hungry neurosurgeons caused the threshold for surgical intervention to drop.

Hospitals play a similar game. Bed capacity, not medical necessity, is the most important factor influencing hospital utilization. Applying a similar economic model to the automobile industry would suggest that if Ford had only manufactured more Edsels, they would have been more popular. We have literally hundreds of hospitals that aren't needed given current levels of need, thereby fostering redundant services that consume precious resources needed elsewhere. Richard D. Lamm, former governor of Colorado and current director of the Center for Public Policy and Contemporary Issues at the University of Denver, remarks, "The most health-producing ethical decision many American hospitals could make would be to close their doors or merge."[18]

Historically, in America, the more plentiful healthcare becomes, the more expensive it gets. In 1991, for example, Broward County, Florida, had nineteen physician-owned magnetic resonance imaging (MRI) machines while Baltimore County, Maryland, had only one; yet the cost of an

MRI scan in Broward County was almost twice that in Baltimore.[19] Interestingly, the additional Florida procedures were performed almost entirely on patients with private health insurance. Steven R. Eastaugh, author of *Health Economics: Efficiency, Quality and Equity*, explains this phenomenon: "Physicians will still make a target income by searching for frill markets catering to consumer fantasies. This may be true for non-insured services, catering to Yuppie boutique medicine." For example, the marketing value of prenatal ultrasound has been exploited by physicians, some of whom perform sonographic evaluations for the sole purpose of providing video-taped souvenirs. But this may soon be a thing of the past. The Food and Drug Administration is investigating a growing industry that performs obstetric ultrasounds for entertainment rather than medical purposes. Complete with voice-over narration, background music, and close-up views of the fetal face and other body parts, these souvenirs cost up to $250 each. According to Joan Baker of the Society of Diagnostic Medical Sonographers, mothers undergoing non-medical, "keepsake" sonograms assume they'll be told if something is wrong when in truth, the technicians may not be trained to recognize fetal abnormalities.[20]

As mentioned earlier, a premium is also placed on innovation and high technology, irrespective of efficacy. The expense is simply passed on to patients or their insurers. A recently published magazine article which featured a private prenatal clinic exemplifies the attitude that pervades contemporary obstetrics:[21]

> "A healthcare team committed to providing the very best and latest."
> "We have an ultrasound machine here in our office for our patients' convenience. . . . We give each of our patients a video of their ultrasound."
> "New and innovative procedures and techniques . . . with the highest level of care."
> "Comfortable, feminine, attractively decorated office."

In a healthcare system operating in a true market economy, the growing supply of obstetricians would eventually drive down the physician component of prenatal care expenses. Instead, every new doctor brings with him or her $400,000 of additional expense to the healthcare budget.[22] As with all other aspects of medicine, obstetrical expenses are not controlled by market demand.[23-26] Despite the flood of new obstetricians that enter practice each year, prenatal care costs have not decreased as any overabundant commodity would in any other market. To make matters worse, many obstetricians have historically been less inclined to accept low-paying (i.e., Medicaid) mothers into their practices.

A Poverty of Riches

Despite the oversupply of medical specialists, obstetricians aren't exactly fanning out over the countryside to provide prenatal care for one and all. It doesn't even appear that they are taking care of mothers at highest risk for complications in many cases. Even though rural mothers tend to be at higher risk for pregnancy-related problems, obstetricians continue to cluster in already over-served metropolitan areas where they load their practices with relatively trouble-free, low-risk patients. For example, a fourteen-state survey conducted by the Institute of Medicine found that 252 counties within those states had no obstetric care providers.[27] Likewise, a 1991 study conducted in Indiana found that only 30 percent of that state's rural counties had adequate numbers of obstetric care providers, and a 1996 study found that seventy-nine of ninety-nine Iowa counties had no obstetricians.[28, 29] Of the 160 obstetricians providing prenatal care in the remaining twenty counties, 157 resided in the eighteen most populous counties (which contained 42 percent of Iowa's population). Thus, the assumption that obstetricians are able and willing to tackle the problems for which they are trained appears to be incorrect.

To illustrate the mismatch between mothers' needs and the care they actually receive, Dr. Sharon Dobie at the University of Washington studied over 14,000 pregnant women only to find that urban obstetricians—those with the greatest amount of specialty training and the easiest access to the most sophisticated facilities—had the fewest patients classified as high risk.[30] On the other hand, rural family practitioners had the greatest proportion of women with high-risk pregnancies. While it is possible that pregnant women at highest risk are eventually referred to obstetricians after their high-risk status is recognized, the reality is that most rural women are covered by Medicaid programs and have limited mobility or motivation to travel long distances for specialized prenatal care. This finding is supported by the low referral rates noted in Dr. Dobie's study.

In another study, Dr. Eugene R. Declercq at Boston University compared the medical characteristics of mothers receiving care from hospital-based midwives against the national average, finding risk profiles that were similar or higher among midwife patients:[31]

Problem	Midwife Patients (%)	All U.S. Births (%)*
Anemia	37.1	19.1
Prior low-birthweight baby	16.9	14.4
Genital herpes	9.3	8.1
Heart disease	3.6	3.6
Lung disease	3.4	3.0
Kidney disease	5.5	2.7

* More than 85% of all U.S. births receive prenatal care from obstetricians.
Reprinted by permission of Blackwell Science, Inc., from E. R. Declercq. "Midwifery Care and Medical Complications: The Role of Risk Screening." *Birth* 2(June 1995)68.

In Arizona, rural women were also more likely than their urban counterparts to have medical complications:[32, 33]

Pregnancy Complications in Arizona *

	1980	1990	1995
Urban (%)	53.9	64.6	70.8
Rural (%)	63.6	72.7	73

* percentage of low-birthweight births
Reprinted with permission of the Arizona Department of Health Services, from J. C. Gersten, C. K. Mrela. *Closing the Decade: Arizona Health Status and Vital Statistics, 1980–1989* (Phoenix: Arizona Department of Health Services, 1990) and from C. K. Mrela. *Arizona Health Status and Vital Statistics, 1995* (Phoenix: Arizona Department of Health Services, 1996).

Through the decade of the 1980s and well into the '90s, the low-birthweight rate for rural Arizona babies was also generally higher than for urban babies:[34, 35]

Low-Birthweight Babies in Arizona

	1980	1990	1995
Urban (%)	6.1	6.4	6.7
Rural (%)	6.3	6.9	7.3

Reprinted with permission of the Arizona Department of Health Services, from J. C. Gersten, C. K. Mrela. *Closing the Decade: Arizona Health Status and Vital Statistics, 1980–1989* (Phoenix: Arizona Department of Health Services, 1990) and from C. K. Mrela. *Arizona Health Status and Vital Statistics, 1995* (Phoenix: Arizona Department of Health Services, 1996).

Nevertheless, the use of nurse-midwives in the high risk rural population of Arizona was 2.4-times more common than in urban areas. Like Dr. Dobie in Washington, the Arizona Department of Health Services attributed this 67 situation to "the shortage of physicians with obstetrical practices in many rural regions."[36]

Expanded Eligibility

Influenced by obstetric experts, Congress initially perceived infant mortality as a problem related to the insufficient availability of prenatal care.[37] Further influenced by the findings of the Institute of Medicine's Committee to Study the Prevention of Low Birthweight which suggested that improving access to early prenatal care for low-income mothers would reduce the rate of low-birthweight infants, Congress conceptualized financial barriers as the single greatest impediment to adequate prenatal care.[38] Expanding Medicaid eligibility became the contemporary strategy for achieving equity in this area. However, scrutiny of the effects of this policy reveals that expanded eligibility alone hasn't provided consistent improvements in pregnancy outcomes.

Although some published data would suggest that reduced Medicaid funding may adversely impact pregnancy outcomes of low-income mothers, the available data reveals that the converse is not necessarily true and suggests that noneconomic issues may influence pregnancy outcomes to a greater degree than previously thought. To illustrate, Dr. Paula Braveman at the University of California in San Francisco found that despite boosting California Medicaid eligibility to 200 percent of the federal poverty level, access to prenatal care was still limited for mothers in this economic group.[39] Other researchers also have found that Medicaid coverage alone may be insufficient for overcoming the many risks associated with low socioeconomic status. For example, when Dr. Joyce M. Piper at Vanderbilt University evaluated the effect of a 1985 Tennessee Medicaid regulatory change that expanded eligibility, she found no improvements in the use of early prenatal care, nor in the rates of low-birthweight or neonatal death.[40] Dr. Piper concluded that, "While in theory expansion of maternal Medicaid enrollment should improve the rates of early prenatal care utilization, there is little research to support the contention that Medicaid coverage alone will have this effect." Likewise, Dr. Jennifer S. Haas of Harvard University assessed the impact of liberalized healthcare coverage to uninsured Massachusetts mothers with incomes below 185 percent of the federal poverty level, finding that the number of women receiving satisfactory prenatal care actually declined.[41] In addition, there was no statewide change in the overall incidence of adverse

68   birth outcomes, suggesting that expanded economic access to prenatal care alone does not necessarily benefit low-income mothers. At the end of her report, Dr. Haas concluded, "Although expanding health coverage may remove the financial barrier to seek care, it may not address other factors that limit access to prenatal care or contribute to poor birth outcomes. A reduction in the high rates of adverse neonatal outcomes may require interventions that address these as well."

In Washington state in the early 1990s, Medicaid eligibility was expanded to 185 percent of the federal poverty level; the prenatal services offered were enhanced (case management, nutritional and psychological counseling, health education, and home visits); and physician reimbursement was increased from $750 to $1,200 per patient without producing statistically significant reductions in Washington's low-birthweight rate.[42] Over the same period in Colorado, Medicaid eligibility was increased to 133 percent of the federal poverty level and physician reimbursement was increased from $510 to $961 per patient without statistically significant improvements in that state's low-birthweight rate.[43] Only when Washington's low-birthweight rate was compared to Colorado's (an apples-to-oranges comparison) was a significant improvement in the low-birthweight rate found—an improvement attributed to Washington state's enhanced prenatal services. Barely mentioned in the report was the fact that low-birthweight rates were unchanged among women with a history of prior premature birth, nor were the researchers able to identify which aspects of the enhanced services spelled the difference for Washington's babies.

Likewise, in California in the early 1990s, enhanced prenatal care was offered as a way to improve pregnancy outcomes.[44] All women with incomes less than 200 percent of the federal poverty level were eligible for prenatal care which included nutritional counseling, social workers, and health education. For each woman, an individualized care plan was developed which outlined and coordinated the support services she was to receive. In addition, prenatal care providers were paid up to $261 extra for each patient who achieved certain predetermined milestones of care during her pregnancy. When the program was evaluated, however, it was found that the rate of low birthweight among those receiving enhanced services was no different than for women receiving routine Medicaid prenatal care. Significantly better outcomes were noted only among a subgroup of women within the program—those with at least eight prenatal visits. But it is unclear if the improved outcomes in this subgroup were a function of the extra clinic visits or if there was something about the women who chose not to keep their pre- natal clinic appointments (i.e., illness, drugs, etc.) which increased the like- **69** lihood for low birthweight. At least part of the explanation lies in the fact that those who delivered prematurely had no need to return for further vis- its. Yet in the final tally, their low-birthweight children were tied to subopti- mal clinic attendance—a cart-before-the-horse statistical quirk mentioned in chapter 2. Nevertheless, the failure of the California project to produce an overall improvement in the low-birthweight rate is in step with other stud- ies which preceded and followed it.

Counterpoint

It might be noted that prior to expansions in Medicaid eligibility, Aid to Families with Dependent Children (AFDC)—Medicaid recipients were the poorest of our citizens, those at highest risk for low-birthweight babies. Thus, it should not be surprising that the addition of less-impoverished (and presumably, lower-risk) women to Medicaid's roles via expanded eligibility would not result in significant improvements in pregnancy outcomes. In essence, expanded Medicaid eligibility dilutes the overall risk level among Medicaid mothers, thereby reducing the likelihood that a measurable im- provement would be observed.[45]

Rebuttal

However, Dr. James W. Krieger of the University of Washington found that an appreciable number of Medicaid mothers, having gained entry into the prenatal care system, did not participate within it in the same fashion as non- Medicaid patients.[46] Krieger observed that, compared to non-Medicaid mothers, ten times as many Medicaid mothers enrolled in prenatal care dur- ing the last trimester of pregnancy. Is the lack of health insurance really the major barrier to early prenatal care in the inner city? That's the question posed by Dr. Winsome Parchment of the University of Medicine and Den- tistry—New Jersey Medical School.[47] In a study conducted in Newark, New Jersey, Dr. Parchment found that the availability of health insurance be- fore and during pregnancy wasn't associated with the adequacy of prenatal care. Even worse, Parchment noted that 71 percent of the mothers who'd received no prenatal care whatsoever actually had health insurance at the time of delivery.

70   As a matter of fact, there's a considerable portion of women for whom prenatal care is available who choose not to partake. A study of low-income mothers delivering at five hospitals in Detroit found that roughly 40 percent avoided prenatal clinics, instead using emergency rooms and walk-in clinics for their prenatal care.[48] Moreover, 62 percent failed to return for postpartum check-ups. Even free care does not guarantee utilization of medical services as demonstrated by the observation that 10 percent of pregnant military personnel, prisoners, and women enrolled in health maintenance organizations fail to secure adequate prenatal care.[49, 50] This phenomenon is evidenced on a larger scale by the experience of the state of Hawaii.[51, 52] Despite that state's willingness to provide free or low-cost private coverage to virtually all uninsured citizens, a considerable portion of residents do not participate.

The assumption that mothers would seek prenatal care if only they had access to it has not been born out for an appreciable number of pregnant women. Prenatal programs across the United States have even attempted to bribe low-income mothers into better prenatal clinic attendance by offering incentives such as baby clothing, diapers, and gift certificates. Dr. Marilyn P. Laken at Wayne State University in Detroit evaluated the utility of such incentives to increase participation in prenatal care.[53] In her study, one group of Medicaid-eligible women was given monetary rewards for each prenatal visit attended while another group received no special inducements. Dr. Laken found that incentives had no impact on the number of kept prenatal appointments, postpartum check-up attendance, or the level of maternal satisfaction.

Improved access to prenatal care has brought unimpressive results because we've improved access to a system that doesn't work. Likewise, intensifying the levels of prenatal care has failed to reduce prematurity because we've intensified something that's fundamentally ineffectual against it. In any other industry, ineffective products are taken off the market. But in obstetrics, the product is repackaged and pushed harder as if through sheer will it can be rendered more effective. By analogy, it's as if our leaders had ordained that every American household be provided with a refrigerator without any concern as to whether the homes have electricity to run them or food to place in them. The mere act of providing refrigerators is sufficient because it shows symbolic concern on the part of government. Meanwhile, the only true beneficiaries are refrigerator manufacturers. Access to prenatal care is far less important than the issues of efficacy and maternal motivation. Yet it's the issue of access to prenatal care that persists as a seminal issue in the industry of women's health.

The Primary Care Scam

In contrast to the fanfare and attention surrounding prenatal care in the United States, non-pregnant women are nearly invisible to prenatal researchers and policymakers. Virtually all strategies for improving pregnancy outcomes—however unsuccessful—have been confined to the prenatal period, essentially prioritizing fetal interests ahead of maternal interests. In many arenas, the health of reproductive-age women is considered only to the degree that it affects their babies—some healthcare plans historically only provided coverage to women while they were pregnant. As Dr. Paul H. Wise at Harvard University notes, "We must recognize that, in some large measure, problems with infant ill health are a legacy of women's ill health generally. . . . An expanded commitment to women's health would help transform prenatal care from the first component of child healthcare to merely one component . . . of women's healthcare across a lifetime."[54]

One way to fulfill Dr. Wise's recommendations is to facilitate women's access to general healthcare services. Indeed, the growing trend away from medical specialists is a welcome development in American healthcare. Specialists take longer to train, charge more for their services, and have historically been less inclined to care for indigent patients or to reside in rural areas. Unlike generalists (i.e., primary care providers), specialists devote themselves to more isolated or esoteric aspects of medicine and tend to ignore the overall health of their patients.

Since 1965, the federal government has subsidized medical education in the United States. Fitzhugh Mullan at the U.S. Bureau of Health Professionals estimates that the government invested over $70,000 for every medical resident in training during 1992.[55] But the number of specialty residency positions is determined by a process that gives no consideration to the number of specialists actually needed by society. The result is a physician workforce whose ranks are swollen by factors that have little to do with the healthcare needs of Americans. According to Dr. John E. Wennberg of Dartmouth University, "The motivations that determine the size of residency programs often concern prestige status among educational institutions, the needs of the directors of the various residency programs and the priceless advantage of the night and weekend coverage that a house staff (i.e., residents) offers the senior staff."[56] The current number of specialists in the United States is more than adequate to meet the specialty healthcare needs of our nation. Indeed, Dr. Wennberg has found that physician excess already exists across the board in America: Pathology, 3.1-fold excess; Neurosurgery, 2.5-fold excess; Anesthesia, 2.0-fold excess; Radiology, 1.5-fold excess and OB/GYN, 1.2-fold excess.[57, 58]

The Association of American Medical Colleges acknowledges that we can no longer defend the inordinate number of medical specialists that are trained each year in the United States.[59] Likewise, the Council on Graduate Medical Education has urged Congress to set limits on the number of medical students and residents so as to achieve a better fit between our nation's needs and the number and distribution of doctors.[60]

As a result of initiatives in the public and private sectors, healthcare dollars for specialists are in ever shorter supply. Unfortunately, the emphasis on general medical care has fostered cynical attempts by some specialists to have their fields designated as primary care, thereby assuring ongoing access to patients. The American College of Obstetricians and Gynecologists (ACOG), for example, now maintains that obstetricians are primary care physicians for women. This tactic was undertaken in response to federal policymakers' proposals that denied obstetricians primary care status. With the help of lobbying from a variety of sources, President Clinton's original proposal was altered to include obstetricians.[61, 62] By promoting their position with the Clinton Administration, obstetricians will continue to be subsidized by federal funds at a rate that will oversupply us with obstetricians that we don't need and that the market won't support. In the words of Dr. David Redwine, an Oregon obstetrician, "In trying to remake themselves as primary care doctors, they try to portray the effort as a proactive, taking-the-bull-by-the-horns approach. It's not. It's a reaction—an unfortunate reaction to crass economics."[63]

That obstetrics is not a primary care specialty is a notion shared by the American Academy of Family Physicians, the American Association of Medical Colleges, the Congressional Committee on Graduate Medical Education, and the Institute of Medicine.[64] At its heart, obstetrics and gynecology is a surgical specialty (unlike pediatrics, family practice, or internal medicine). Based upon obstetricians' level of reimbursement, the maldistribution of obstetricians into urban areas and the huge differences in malpractice insurance premiums compared to real primary care providers, obstetricians can never be considered true primary care providers. Moreover, the training of obste-

72

tricians has historically de-emphasized those aspects of women's health which do not directly relate to pregnancy or gynecology. Indeed, the proportion of obstetricians who can meaningfully interpret basic tests such as electrocardiograms is alarmingly low. To foist obstetrics and gynecology upon American women as a form of primary healthcare serves no one but obstetricians as they secure their share of a shrinking economic pool and federal funding for their academic programs. If this tactic is accepted by American women, can it be long before urologists claim primary care status for American men?

Dr. Sheilah Leader reviewed data from three national surveys of members of the American College of Obstetricians and Gynecologists: among nearly 1,300 obstetricians, less than half considered themselves primary care providers.[65] Noting that nearly 40 percent of ACOG members do not provide primary care, Dr. Ralph W. Hale of the American College of Obstetricians and Gynecologists commented indirectly on the oversupply of obstetricians: "Certainly some of our members will not choose to do primary care and will practice by referrals; others will limit their practice to specific subspecialty areas. There is nothing wrong with this; it simply reflects the opportunities available."

Genuine primary care providers don't have the luxury of choosing to practice primary care as Dr. Hale asserts obstetricians do. Their specialty is primary care. The fact that obstetricians have historically been primary care providers for a considerable number of American women does not mean that American women have been receiving genuine primary care; rather, it demonstrates yet another example of the historic, widespread mismatch between the level of care that women need and what they actually receive.

Of the nine most common health screening and diagnostic services provided in this country (in descending order of their frequency: blood pressure analysis, urinalysis, Pap smear, visual acuity, cholesterol, mammogram, electrocardiogram, chest X-ray, and throat culture), none require the specific services of an obstetrician. Indeed, five of these services (urinalysis, cholesterol, mammogram, electrocardiogram and chest X-ray) aren't even performed by physicians; they're merely ordered by physicians.

The newfound interest by the specialty of obstetrics and gynecology in primary care is more an example of ingenuity than altruism. That obstetrics and gynecology should provide genuine primary care was first recommended over twenty years ago, restated in 1980 and again in 1986 with almost no concomitant effort by ACOG to promote or ensure that real primary care was being provided, until the specter of economic losses was raised in 1992 by federal policymakers who proposed that the specialty be excluded from primary care status.[66-68] In response, the curriculum for American OB/GYN residents was modified in 1996 so as to give each trainee six months of primary care experience. In order to achieve this, however, the residents' training in OB/GYN was cut by six months despite concerns that the residents' clinical and surgical skills would be compromised in order to accommodate the primary care training.[69, 70] Moreover, primary care physicians have expressed concerns that six months of primary care are insufficient to allow mastery of the subject. Thus, it is feared that new obstetricians will matriculate with diluted training in their own specialty and inadequate experience in primary care when the first batch of residents to have been trained under the new arrangement enters the market in the year 2000.

To categorize the specialty of obstetrics and gynecology as primary care is a mistake that will ultimately compromise the well-being of women and produce a glut of obstetricians. Optimizing the health of women, pregnant or otherwise, entails more than the care of their reproductive organs and is better accomplished by non-obstetricians. Moreover, basic gynecologic care is already being provided in excellent fashion by nurse-midwives and family practitioners and does not require an expensive, extensive four-year obstetrics and gynecology residency.

The argument has been posited by the American College of Obstetricians and Gynecologists that obstetricians should be considered primary care providers because many women's only contact with the medical system is through obstetricians. While this notion has been successfully promoted to the Clinton Administration, it leaves women's primary healthcare in the hands of specialists who generally underserve rural, poor, and minority women to a greater extent than do family practitioners, internists, and certified nurse-midwives.[71]

Have most obstetricians even been trained to provide primary care to women? Dr. Marc L. Rivo with the Council on Graduate Medical Education conducted a study to determine the extent to which residency training programs prepare their young physicians for primary care.[72] Dr. Rivo determined the extent to which each residency's requirements fulfilled sixty primary care training objectives. Rivo found that almost all objectives were met by family practice (95 percent), internal medicine (91 percent) and pediatrics (91 percent), compared to obstetrics and gynecology (47 percent). Based on his findings, Dr. Rivo concluded that only family practice, internal medicine, and pediatric training programs prepare their residents in the "broad competencies" required for the primary care of patients. Indeed, during a survey of Michigan obstetricians, 74 percent stated that they had   **75** not received the necessary residency training to provide primary care. Coincident with the convenient appearance of primary care courses for practicing obstetricians is the publication of the new ACOG journal *Primary Care Update for OB/GYN's*. Relative to the journal *Obstetrics and Gynecology* (which contains more than twenty-five articles, 150–200 pages per month), the bimonthly *Primary Care Update for OB/GYN's* (with less than 10 articles, fewer than 50 pages per month) reveals ACOG's venture into primary care to be window-dressing. Meanwhile, ACOG is preparing to unveil yet another OB/GYN subspecialty ("urogynecology")—a clear move towards further specialization and away from the province of primary care to which ACOG has stridently claimed obstetricians belong.

A "Primary" Example

Let's examine an important issue for which primary care providers must be well-versed: domestic violence. Physical abuse is the single most common cause of injury to American women. Indeed, 30 percent of women visiting hospital emergency rooms do so because of domestic violence.[73, 74] The most conservative research data regarding its incidence estimates that 4 percent of our nation's women are victims of battering. During pregnancy, domestic violence is associated with a host of prenatal complications, including prematurity.

Having claimed the mantle of primary healthcare providers for women, how are obstetricians dealing with domestic violence? Most don't even know it exists. A nationwide study of obstetricians conducted by Dr. Linda R. Chambliss at Maricopa County Medical Center in Phoenix found that only 5 percent of obstetricians estimated the prevalence of battering at anywhere near the rates reported in national surveys.[75] Routine screening of all women for domestic violence has been recommended by the American College of Obstetricians and Gynecologists (ACOG) for over a decade. Even so, a study by Deborah L. Horan at ACOG found that only about four out of every ten pregnant women were routinely screened for the problem.[76] To make matters worse, half of obstetrics and gynecology residency directors believe that the problem is better handled by others.

What We Can Do about It: Step Three

1. Regionalization Should Be Preserved

Regionalization of perinatal and neonatal care is associated with better outcomes while deregionalization is associated with less optimal ones. Moreover, the duplication of services that deregionalization inevitably produces results in needless expense and dilution of clinical experience vital to maintaining the expertise that high risk personnel require for optimal maternal and fetal outcomes. The distribution of perinatal and neonatal services should be based on the characteristics of a given region as determined by unbiased perinatal and neonatal experts who have no political or economic stake in a given region. Regionalization must never be based upon the local self-interests of physicians or hospital administrators who seek greater market penetration within an established region. Prurient economic interests must never take precedence over the medical interests of mother and child. If perinatal and neonatal organizations cannot halt the trend, state and federal regulation should be enacted to prevent further deregionalization.

To ensure that mothers don't fall victim to a process that's economically rather than medically driven, they should be asking certain questions when acute pregnancy complications arise:

QUESTIONS FOR THE OBSTETRICIAN

- How often do you treat patients with my particular complication?
- Do you have special training or expertise for my problem?
- Is there someone in the area with more expertise?
- Do the doctors who take call for you have the same level of expertise that you do?

Upon completing their training, most obstetricians enter private practice where, over the years, many become isolated from the care of high-risk pregnancies. Less frequent contact with complicated patients does not foster the competence that acute, high-risk cases deserve. Remember, practice makes perfect. An obstetrician who possessed expertise in a particular pregnancy complication in 1970 or 1980 may not have maintained his or her expertise over the ensuing years of low-risk patient care at outpost hospitals. Therefore, it's important to know how practiced one's obstetrician is with serious pregnancy problems—few doctors are likely to volunteer the information.

Obstetricians frequently participate with their peers in a rotating night-time on-call pool. By doing so, obstetricians can avoid being on-call twenty-four hours a day, seven days a week—an emotionally and physically draining endeavor. In a sufficiently large pool, obstetricians' frequency of night-call can fall to one night per week or less. However, when he/she is on call, his/her patient load can easily exceed one hundred patients. While most of the patients that the "on-call" physician covers do not require medical service, the point is that on-call obstetricians frequently know nothing about the patients for whom they're responsible. On any given night, women in labor have a significant likelihood that they'll be delivered by someone other than their own obstetrician. While patients' own obstetricians may be quite adept at diagnosing pregnancy problems and may be current regarding the care of such problems, their on-call peers may not.

QUESTIONS ABOUT THE HOSPITAL

- Is there a higher-level facility in the region from which I or my baby might benefit?
- What is the average number of babies in the neonatal intensive care unit at this hospital?
- What is the lowest gestational age for which this hospital's nursery routinely cares?

The younger or sicker a baby is, the higher level of care it will need. The highest level of care will be found at a regional center. Period. Don't accept suggestions that outpost hospitals are "just as good as" regional centers. They aren't. Especially for newborns younger than thirty-two to thirty-four weeks gestation at delivery, the clinical expertise and technical abilities provided by regional level III centers cannot be matched by outpost institutions. As we have seen, premature babies at outpost centers are at greater risk for suboptimal outcomes when compared to babies at level III centers. When complications arise, a mother should request her hospital's most recent neonatal survival statistics. A quick review will not only provide survival rates, it will reveal the actual number of babies at each gestational age that that institution has treated during a given year. Moreover, it will allow for meaningful comparison with other facilities in the region. Beware of hospitals that cannot readily produce their newborn statistics. If uncertainty persists, mothers should request a consultation with the hospital's neonatologist and/or maternal-fetal specialist to identify the appropriate institutional setting. Absence of twenty-four-hour in-hospital access to these specialists should alert you to the likelihood that you aren't at a level III center. Not all situations will require referral to a regional center. But in a changing economic environment, mothers must remain mindful of the fact that some doctors will retain patients who have problems that are out of their usual range of clinical practice.

2. Genuine Primary Care Is a Must

Primary care should be accessible to women. But to repackage obstetrics as primary care promotes inadequate overall healthcare for women. Rather than changing the categorization of obstetricians, we should change the mindset of policymakers and patients. Obstetricians' attempt to be proclaimed primary care providers is an economically driven ploy that must be resisted. To depend entirely upon obstetricians to provide total healthcare for women is a mistake. Women's health screening and maintenance will be more comprehensive, ubiquitous, and economical when the primary care of essentially healthy women is left to genuine primary care providers. Taxpayers pay for the overwhelming majority of medical education in this nation, contributing twenty-five billion dollars to train many professionals that we simply don't need. Therefore, prenatal care reform should include obstetric workforce reform.

The next few years will see a glut of obstetricians whose training has been subsidized by taxpayer dollars that feed a system which fosters inaccessibility to healthcare providers. According to Dr. John E. Wennberg at Dartmouth University, "One of the most persistent and dysfunctional health policy myths is the belief that the best way to get physicians to locate in underserved areas is to produce such an excess in supply that physicians will move there because they cannot survive economically elsewhere."[77] At present, obstetrics and gynecology training programs frequently petition the American Board of Obstetricians and Gynecologists for permission to increase the number of residents in training—a maneuver designed to alleviate the workload of the institution and not the anticipated need for obstetricians in practice. For most programs to be in step with future national needs, they would need to reduce the number of residents in training immediately—some training programs should be closed. Since many obstetrics and gynecology residencies exist simply to provide care for a given community's indigent maternity population, loss of such programs will require that other arrangements be made for the care of these mothers. Funds presently spent for local residency programs could instead be spent for prenatal care with private practice physicians, or preferably, nurse-midwives. However, this discussion may soon be rendered moot: rumblings from the U.S. House of Representative's Ways and Means Committee suggest that the federal government may stop paying for graduate medical education in the coming years.[78]

3. Obstetric Workforce Reform

SPLIT OBSTETRICS AND GYNECOLOGY INTO TWO SEPARATE
MEDICAL SPECIALTIES

Earlier this century, obstetrics was a separate medical specialty from gynecology. By mid-century, however, all American residency programs had consolidated into the specialty as we presently know it. On the surface, combining obstetrics and gynecology would seem to make sense. Both specialties involve the healthcare of women and both demand a thorough understanding of female anatomy and physiology. To have a single healthcare provider well versed in both fields appears to be a logical notion that would promote continuity of care for women. Besides, there are situations where an obstetric condition may impact a woman's gynecologic health and vice versa. But there are also significant differences between the two fields regarding the nature of care, risk factors, and patient types.

The essential difference between obstetric and gynecologic patients is, obviously, that obstetric patients are pregnant. A variety of anatomic and physiologic changes occur during pregnancy that set pregnant women apart from their non-pregnant peers. Equally important is the fact that pregnancy is a normal condition whereas gynecology is a specialty devoted to problems of the female reproductive tract. Although gynecology also provides some preventive healthcare for women, it's essentially a specialty devoted to disease. Another difference between obstetric and gynecologic patients involves the age and health of the two groups. The incidence of cancer and heart disease is significantly lower among women of reproductive age. Routine obstetric care involves the management of a natural process in women who tend to be young and healthy whereas gynecology provides care for women who frequently have multiple medical problems and are older. In fact, many gynecologic patients are elderly and/or moribund, making an understanding of gerontologic medicine necessary for the gynecologist. As will be mentioned later, many obstetricians build their practice on obstetrics with the hope that it will evolve into a practice that's largely gynecology-based. By separating the two specialties, only those who intend to provide obstetrical services for the entirety of their career will pursue obstetric training.

TRAIN PROSPECTIVE OBSTETRICIANS TO BE MATERNAL-FETAL (HIGH-RISK) SPECIALISTS

At present, obstetrics and gynecology is subdivided into three subspecialties: oncology(cancer), endocrine/infertility, and maternal-fetal medicine (high-risk pregnancy). Upon completion of a four-year residency in general obstetrics, one may elect to pursue a two- to three-year fellowship for training in one of the subspecialty fields, thereby achieving special competence and expertise. In general, however, only a small fraction of obstetricians pursue subspecialty training. Unable to provide the high-risk expertise that a changed paradigm and hostile medicolegal climate demand, yet unable to provide low-risk prenatal care that's affordable and affords ample time for each mother, the general obstetrician has become outmoded. Ongoing reliance upon a system of prenatal care that's obstetrician-based will steadily drive prenatal care costs higher and will further promote the factory style of prenatal care that many obstetricians already provide (chapter 4). But more importantly, it won't improve our nation's embarrassing status in the world regarding prematurity and low birthweight. To respond to the present state of affairs in American prenatal care, the training process of American obstetricians should be changed. As mentioned previously, issues to be considered before initiating any changes in obstetric residency programs should include the following:

- The anticipated excess of obstetricians that the next decade will bring.
- The superfluous role that obstetricians play relative to the roles of certified nurse-midwives and maternal-fetal specialists (chapter 4).
- A modification that takes these issues into consideration would do away with general obstetrics as we presently know it. Instead of a four-year training program as it now exists, an additional two to three years of training should be required. The first four years of training would be similar to how it currently exists, with emphasis in general obstetrics and some gynecology. The next two or three years would be dedicated solely to obstetrics, especially high-risk pregnancy. In essence, an obstetrics residency would be almost indistinguishable from the curriculum currently pursued by maternal-fetal specialists. When coupled with the division of obstetrics and gynecology into

separate specialties, the end result would be that all obstetricians would be maternal-fetal specialists and general obstetrics would eventually cease to exist. A new gynecology residency, with its reduced exposure to obstetrics, would be able to provide ample time for training in primary care, effectively transforming gynecologists into genuine primary care providers for women.

A considerable number of high-risk mothers live in rural areas—the very place where obstetricians are in shortest supply. There are a variety of ways that rural, high-risk mothers could receive appropriate levels of care. The most reasonable option is for maternal-fetal specialists to provide care at a central clinic for a given rural area on a regular basis. Itinerant maternal-fetal specialists could facilitate access to appropriate levels of prenatal care, reduce unnecessary transport of mothers, and allow earlier intervention for mothers who might not have the resources or desire to travel long distances to a perinatal center until their pregnancy complications have become more obvious or advanced.

4. The Stakeholders

Obstetricians

The Perception of Pregnancy as a Disease

Imagine what would happen if one day the lifeguard at the community swimming pool assumed that every person splashing around in his pool were drowning? In this scenario, would every swimmer plucked from the water really have been saved? Besides making a nuisance of himself, the lifeguard might actually cause harm with his unnecessary interventions. The situation is nearly identical to what many American mothers experience with prenatal care.

Although a pregnant woman will undergo many anatomic and physiologic changes over the course of gestation, she's nevertheless a healthy person. Most pregnancies are, medically speaking, uneventful affairs. Nevertheless, contemporary obstetrics has created a context wherein mothers are considered sick until proven otherwise. According to Dr. Bruce Flamm at the University of California in Riverside, "Obstetricians have always been trained to believe that pregnancy and labor are disasters waiting to happen. That means that obstetricians tend to use more medical interventions and pay less attention to the emotional concerns of women."[1] Draping pregnancy with a medical imperative allows us to avoid discussions regarding the necessity or utility of prenatal care. It's a medical matter and that's that. Clearly, pregnancy is a watershed event in the life of a family. It's a major change, a transition fraught with uncertainty, but it isn't a medical emergency. Consequently, a normal condition has been unnecessarily medicalized. Pregnant women thereby enter into a system from which the majority receive no real benefit.

Many improvements in American pregnancy outcomes have been mistakenly ascribed to prenatal care, erroneously bolstering our faith in its effectiveness. Earlier this century, for example, the benefit that medical science afforded mothers was a manifestation of what the general public as a whole enjoyed. Obstetrics had very little to do with early improvements in maternal and child health. Most of the progress made in this realm was accomplished by low-tech strategies: child-spacing, housing, hygiene, and nutrition.[2, 3] Maternal mortality rates began to drop well before the creation of antibiotics, blood banks, or obstetric committees on maternal mortality rates.[4] Nevertheless, obstetricians assimilated a system of care indistinguishable from that found in large medical institutions. The rigid regimens of prenatal and postpartum care inherent in an institutionalized approach—reinforced by the post-World War II baby boom when the surging pregnancy rate stressed obstetric facilities—still persist in many regions of the country today.[5]

Medicalization Makes Prenatal Care More Expensive

The use of obstetricians for the delivery of prenatal care is an immensely inefficient and expensive endeavor. To become an obstetrician, an individual must complete four years of college (with a heavy science emphasis), four years of medical school and four years of residency training. At the end of the process, the new obstetrician is typically in his/her thirties, in debt, and more than ready for the generous income and comfortable lifestyle that his/her dedication and hard work have earned. Indeed, the American Medical Association's Socioeconomic Monitoring System noted that the median net income for American obstetricians in 1993 was $200,000 a year.[6]

New obstetricians generally build their practice by seeing a large number of pregnant women in the hopes that these patients will return later in life for their gynecologic needs. In essence, obstetrics is what sustains a young obstetrician's practice, but it's gynecology, where the least medicolegal risk exists, that most prefer to practice. Moreover, most gynecologic problems can be managed during office hours as compared to the round-the-clock demands of obstetrics. Many seek to curtail the obstetric aspect of their practice as soon as the gynecologic component can support them—cursory review of the Yellow Pages in any American city will show the strong emphasis that most obstetricians place upon the non-obstetric aspects of their practice (infertility, endometriosis, premenstrual syndrome, family planning, cancer surgery, laser surgery, etc.).

How do high-tech providers of prenatal care such as obstetricians stack up against low-tech nurse-midwives? The available information would suggest that care provided by obstetricians to low-risk pregnant women is no better than that provided by nurse-midwives, except that it's more expensive. But how much more expensive are obstetricians? To answer the question, Dr. Deborah Oakley at the University of Michigan analyzed the professional fees and hospital charges generated by obstetricians and compared them to those of nurse-midwives. Dr. Oakley found that nurse-midwives are a bargain: on average, they were over $1,300 cheaper for total maternity care.[7] If we convert the professional fees of obstetricians and nurse-midwives into hourly wages, the cost differences become even more striking, given that nurse-midwives tend to spend more time with their patients than do obstetricians.

While the actual meaning of the term "quality" is subject to interpretation, the available evidence suggests that in terms of gestational age and birthweight, the quality of prenatal care provided by nurse-midwives to low-risk mothers is equivalent to that provided by obstetricians. In general, quality is considered high when pregnancy outcome is optimal and patient satisfaction is high. With the growing recognition that care provided to low-risk mothers by nurse-midwives generally achieves similar pregnancy outcomes at lower cost, one could argue that, dollar for dollar, higher overall quality is provided by midwives. Moreover, evidence to be considered later suggests that patient satisfaction among women cared for by certified nurse-midwives is frequently higher than that among mothers receiving prenatal care from obstetricians, thereby tipping the quality scale even further in favor of nurse-midwives. Obstetricians are doing nothing wrong when they staff, equip, and decorate their office(s) generously. As with any other subculture, one must keep up with the Joneses. The obstetrician whose office is indistinguishable from a boutique is marketing himself by giving the customer what he thinks she wants. The costs of such amenities are simply passed along to patients. Moreover, the expense that medical malpractice premiums generate (on average, $30,000 to $80,000 per year) can easily push the annual overhead for even a small obstetrics practice well beyond $100,000. For example, according to Lauren M. Walker, senior associate editor for Medical Economics, the median tax-deductible practice expenses for American obstetricians in 1993 was over $150,000.[8] A 1997 survey of nearly 3,800 doctors found that the mean overhead costs for obstetrics was almost $300,000 per year.[9]

Thus, prenatal care provided by obstetricians has a sizable portion of built-in costs. In order for the obstetrician to meet these expenses, a relatively large number of patients must be seen. Obviously, as a practice grows, more demands are placed upon the obstetrician. The end result is that the obstetrician has less time for any given mother. Ancillary staff frequently become the primary providers of prenatal care. Meanwhile, expenses mount—not a significant problem in the days of unlimited insurance reimbursement, but a foreboding trend with the move towards managed care.

85

There are countless babies whose lives have been saved by the clinical acumen and quick action of obstetricians. In addition, most ongoing research in the field and many obstetrical breakthroughs may be attributed to obstetricians. But in an environment where cost-effectiveness is the password, obstetricians' built-in expenses may some day price them out of the prenatal market.

Obstetricians as Barriers to Prenatal Care

Impediments to the receipt of prenatal care are frequently portrayed as barriers set between pregnant women and obstetricians. If it weren't for the barriers, according to this logic, women would gladly seek prenatal care and obstetricians would gladly provide it. As we saw in the preceding chapter, however, women don't always seek prenatal care gladly. Unfortunately, it appears that obstetricians don't always gladly provide it, either. A 1985 national survey conducted by the American College of Obstetricians and Gynecologists, for example, found that only six of ten obstetricians who provided prenatal care services provided it for Medicaid women.[10] Likewise, in twenty-six Northern California counties, a 20-percent drop occurred in the number of physicians accepting new Medicaid patients in the early 1990s.[11] Dr. Barbara M. Aved surveyed a small group of Sacramento obstetricians regarding their reluctance to provide care for pregnant Medicaid women.[12] After financial considerations, Medicaid patient characteristics and malpractice concerns were cited most frequently by the obstetricians. Specifically, they considered Medicaid women to be more difficult to care for and to be less compliant. The doctors also cited cultural and socioeconomic differences as well as Medicaid patients' personal hygiene habits as reasons for their reluctance to provide care, considerations which don't exactly put obstetricians in a favorable light. The characterization of Medicaid women as overly litigious may also be unfounded. A study by Dr. Thomas R. Moore of the University of California at San Diego, for example, reviewed over 22,000 hospital records and found that women with private health insurance were twice as likely to sue as publicly funded patients.[13] Additionally, a review of over 31,000 medical records in New York found that poor patients were significantly less likely to file malpractice claims;[14] two other reports found poor patients were no more likely to sue than wealthier cohorts.[15, 16] As such, obstetricians themselves may represent part of the problem when it comes to access to prenatal care for poor women. But as we shall see later in the chapter, the changes wrought by managed care have recently rendered pregnant Medicaid women much more attractive to private practice obstetricians than they used to be—attractive enough, at least, for obstetricians to overlook concerns about culture, hygiene, and litigiousness.

Medicalization May Actually Increase the Risk of Malpractice Claims

Obstetricians receive virtually no formal training in the psychosocial aspects of pregnancy or interpersonal communication. Since most uncomplicated, low-risk pregnancies generally have few problems, a considerable portion of prenatal care involves patient education and reassurance, two things for which many obstetricians have marginal interest and even less time. But because non-obstetricians—especially nurse-midwives—value the psychosocial, interpersonal, and educational aspects of prenatal care, they tend to place greater emphasis upon these issues. As a result, the rapport between a nurse-midwife and her patient is frequently much stronger than that found between an obstetrician and his/her patient.

Not surprisingly, nurse-midwives tend to be better at providing services that depend on communication with patients.[17] A report by the Institute of Medicine suggests that non-physician prenatal care providers tend to relate to their patients in a non-authoritarian manner and to emphasize education, support, and patient satisfaction.[18] As a result, mothers served by nurse-midwives are more likely to keep prenatal care appointments, to follow treatment regimens,[19] and to express fears and anxieties that they feel are too trivial or silly to put to physicians.[20] Additionally, nurse-midwives tend to care for a smaller number of patients, thereby allowing themselves more time to spend with each patient during prenatal care visits.

Frequently, malpractice claims arise not from actual malpractice but in response to poor communication on the part of the caregiver. Several studies illustrate the point: Dr. Gerald B. Hickson at Vanderbilt University in Nashville, Tennessee, analyzed factors that prompted families to file malpractice claims following birth injuries. Dr. Hickson conducted in-depth interviews with Florida families who had filed malpractice claims against obstetricians, finding that most respondents complained about at least one aspect of their interactions with their obstetricians:[21]

- 32 percent felt that their physicians wouldn't talk or answer questions.
- 13 percent believed that their doctors wouldn't listen.
- 48 percent felt that their physicians had misled them.
- 70 percent indicated that they weren't given appropriate prognoses regarding their infants.

In response to the question, "What was wrong with the care you or your child received?," 29 percent of the respondents noted that their physicians were unavailable when needed. To the question, "What exactly prompted you to initiate a claim?," 24 percent stated that their physicians hadn't been completely honest with them. Another 20 percent filed suit simply to find out from their doctors what actually happened. Several other reports indicate that patients and physicians have different expectations about the type and amount of information that should be communicated. Equally concerning is a study by M. L. May which found that patients who filed malpractice claims felt that their doctors didn't care about them personally.[22] Prompted by the results of his study, Dr. Hickson comments, "Some physicians simply fail to appreciate the full extent of patients' informational needs. . . . Physicians still have much to learn about what their patients want to know and how to convey such information effectively."[23] With the premise that patient satisfaction will be improved if the prenatal care provider spends more time with each mother, obstetricians continue to place themselves at risk: the average length of time of a prenatal visit with a nurse-midwife is 23.7 minutes, with a significant portion spent on teaching and counseling.[24] By comparison, the National Ambulatory Medical Center Survey found that most prenatal visits to physicians last ten minutes, with one-third of the visits lasting no longer than five minutes.[25]

The expectation—enshrined in popular opinion—is that obstetricians provide superior care. As such, the likelihood that a woman will sue following a poor pregnancy outcome is generally greater when the care provider is an obstetrician. The prospects are bolstered by the fact that obstetricians generally carry much larger malpractice insurance policies, thereby providing a "deeper pocket" to the plaintiff than does a nurse-midwife. Add to this the fact that women are less satisfied by their obstetricians and the ever shorter lengths of prenatal visits associated with managed care and the potential for malpractice claims increases. It shouldn't be news, therefore, that the incidence of malpractice claims against nurse-midwives is relatively low. Malpractice premiums for nurse-midwives are a fraction of what American obstetricians pay.

88

Medicalization Doesn't Improve Pregnancy Outcomes

During his/her residency, the obstetrician becomes proficient at many aspects of pregnancy. He/she gains experience managing the complex medical problems of high-risk pregnancies, forceps and cesarean deliveries, and a wide range of treatment modalities. The obstetrician is a well-trained specialist. But few, if any, of these skills are necessary to provide conscientious, high-quality prenatal care to the majority of pregnant women. Despite the extensive training that obstetricians receive, there's no evidence that they produce outcomes superior to those whose prenatal care is given by non-obstetricians.[26] In a study performed in Berkeley, California, by Dr. Howard Blanchette, for example, the pregnancy outcomes of women whose prenatal care was provided entirely by certified nurse-midwives was no different than that provided by obstetricians, with the one exception that the nurse-midwife group underwent significantly fewer cesarean deliveries than the obstetrician group.[27] What makes Dr. Blanchette's study particularly impressive is the fact that the mothers receiving prenatal care from certified nurse-midwives had characteristics which placed them at higher risk for poor pregnancy outcomes. Blanchette's findings were virtually duplicated by the experiences of Dr. Theodore W. Loring of Eureka, California,[28] who studied over 2,000 mothers, and Dr. Raymond J. Jennett of Phoenix, Arizona, who studied more than 10,000 patients.[29] Likewise, a report from the United Kingdom cast nurse-midwives in a favorable light. The report compared the pregnancy outcomes of women in England against those in France during a 19-year period.[30] Because both countries possess reliable national statistics and have similar demographic features, comparisons are reasonable. But the two countries differ significantly with regard to how prenatal care is provided. In England, most women receive prenatal care from non-obstetricians, whereas in France, the majority of pregnant women receive prenatal care solely from obstetricians. Nevertheless, the perinatal mortality rates and frequencies of low-birthweight babies and preterm delivery are the same in both countries.

But are nurse-midwives equipped to detect pregnancy problems when they arise? Extremely. The commonly encountered complications of pregnancy are detected by various prenatal laboratory tests (none of which are **89** actually administered by the obstetrician) or via physical examination. What's more, the physical assessment performed at a routine prenatal visit isn't complicated and does not require a physician. No less than eleven studies have demonstrated the effectiveness of prenatal care provided by certified nurse-midwives.[31–41] In South Carolina, a study by Dr. Henry C. Heins, Jr., of the University of South Carolina found that the pregnancy outcomes of women at high risk for premature delivery who received prenatal care from nurse-midwives were indistinguishable from mothers receiving care from obstetricians.[42]

The most recent study to date on the issue of quality was that conducted by Dr. Deborah Oakley at the University of Michigan.[43] Dr. Oakley's work is one of a growing number of studies which sheds light on the quality of care provided by obstetricians and nurse-midwives. In her analysis of nearly 1,200 low-risk mothers, Dr. Oakley uncovered some intriguing findings. Most importantly, Dr. Oakley found no difference between obstetricians and nurse-midwives with regard to prematurity and low birthweight. However, pregnant women receiving care from obstetricians had significantly higher rates of postpartum hemorrhage and major lacerations of their vaginas. Moreover, their babies had significantly more abrasions. Women receiving care from obstetricians were much more likely to undergo cesarean or forceps deliveries. And what of mothers' satisfaction with their care? Using a five-point scale, Dr. Oakley noted that patient satisfaction was significantly higher for women receiving care from nurse-midwives.

Am I saying that midwives are better than obstetricians? Emphatically, no. But for uncomplicated pregnancies (i.e., 70 to 90 percent of all pregnant women), obstetricians can't do any better than midwives do. Indeed, obstetricians are to routine prenatal care what neurosurgeons are to simple headaches: overkill. Economically speaking, midwives are a tremendous bargain. The perception that they're somehow belowstairs when it comes to low-risk prenatal care is incorrect. By any measure—pregnancy outcome, expense, patient satisfaction, time spent with patients—midwives fare as well or better than obstetricians. But even if widespread use of nurse-midwives in America were to produce no change whatsoever in our national pregnancy statistics, American women would still be better off by way of lower costs and more widespread availability of general healthcare providers. Having cornered the market for low-risk pregnancies, obstetricians have abandoned their hold on the complicated patients they were originally trained to treat. As a result, many will gradually find themselves excluded from the prenatal care game: overtrained for low-risk care and underexperienced for the difficult cases they relinquish to maternal-fetal specialists. In an ever-changing healthcare industry, the day is coming when insurance companies will no longer pay obstetricians' fees when equivalent low-risk care can be purchased more inexpensively from midwives. Indeed, many insurers are paying progressively less per patient, a trend with potentially devastating implications for obstetricians.

Counterpoint

One might argue that studies comparing nurse-midwife outcomes against those of obstetricians are biased and misleading for several reasons, the most important one being that in many of the comparison studies, patients in the midwife groups who developed problems were transferred to obstetricians for the remainder of their pregnancies. Thus, these studies virtually guaranteed that the midwife groups would have the healthiest patients and that the obstetrician groups, by virtue of their inheritance of sicker patients, would have worse pregnancy outcomes. The fact that the studies ultimately showed similarly good outcomes for the midwife and obstetrician groups is a testament to the quality of care provided by obstetricians.

Rebuttal

The above criticism is precisely correct. The nurse-midwife groups in some of the studies ultimately took care of less complicated patients, and the more difficult cases were transferred to obstetricians. But this fact does not diminish the utility of nurse-midwife care, whatsoever. Rather, it demonstrates how well a nationwide system based on nurse-midwives might work: low-risk mothers (the vast majority of pregnant women) would be well cared for by nurse-midwives, and more complex pregnancies would be sent to obstetricians. Instead of the current system whereby a pregnant woman's level of risk doesn't necessarily correlate with the level of care she actually receives, the available data supports rather than questions the benefits of a less medicalized system of care for the majority of our nations' pregnant women—a topic discussed in greater detail at the end of the chapter.

Lawyers

The first recorded liability case brought on behalf of a fetus for prenatal injury occurred in 1884, although the Massachusetts Supreme Court refused to recognize the action.[44] Justice Oliver Wendell Holmes based his opinion on the notion that the fetus was part of the mother at the time of injury and that any awards should be recoverable by the mother and not the unborn child. The ruling held sway for sixty years. But in 1946, the District Court for the District of Columbia concluded that a child could recover for negligently induced prenatal injuries. The court found that, "It is but natural justice that a child, if born alive and viable, should be allowed to maintain an action in the courts for injuries wrongfully committed upon its person while in the womb of its mother."[45] In essence, the court found that the duty of obstetricians extends to the child. In New Jersey, Supreme Court Justice Proctor wrote:

> Justice requires that the principle be recognized that a child has a legal right to begin life with a sound mind and body. If the wrongful conduct of another interferes with that right, and it can be established by competent proof that there is a causal connection between the wrongful interference and the harm suffered by the child when born, damages for such harm should be recoverable by the child.[46]

And the rest is history.

Malpractice, Real and Imagined

Although the United States has only 5 percent of the world's population, it possesses 70 to 80 percent of the planet's attorneys.[47] In Japan, there are twenty engineers for every lawyer—here, there are 2.5 lawyers for every engineer.[48] In 1990, according to Dr. Hugh R. K. Barber, one hundred million suits were filed in state courts alone—nearly one for every two Americans.[49] Medicolegal liability has adversely impacted medicine, especially obstetrics and gynecology. While the putative goal of malpractice attorneys has been to improve the quality of medical care, there's little evidence this has actually occurred. American law schools release 40,000 new graduates annually. The legal profession is growing seven times more rapidly than is the general population; between 1970 and 1990, the number of attorneys in this nation more than doubled.[50] In an increasingly crowded field, ever lower thresholds for initiating claims are becoming necessary to ensure lawyers' economic survival. Indeed, some now buy the names of potential clients from agencies that search for "victims."[51]

The present system rewards lawyers for taking routine claims before juries to convince them that the physician and his deep pockets (i.e., malpractice insurance companies) should pay not only for actual harm done to the patient but also for intangible pain and suffering. Working on a contingency basis, lawyers have convinced a sizable portion of the public that they have nothing to lose by pursuing litigation against any perceived wrongdoer. The mentality fostered by personal injury attorneys has encouraged Americans to pursue lawsuits with abandon. Moreover, skyrocketing malpractice awards have encouraged physicians to practice defensive medicine, subjecting patients to unnecessary, sometimes painful or dangerous tests that frequently don't improve outcomes but provide potentially useful evidence that "proper" care was rendered.

Malpractice attorneys aren't the only ones to have profited from the present arrangement. According to Ralph Nader, "The medical malpractice insurance companies have been registering record profits. . . . In 1991, they had a 28- to 29-percent return on net worth, extremely high by comparison with any other industry or most insurance carriers."[52]

Since 1933, tort costs (the costs of defending suits in court, awards to plaintiffs, and administrative overhead) have grown 400-fold, outstripping the growth rate of the Gross National Product by a factor of four.[53] In 1991, tort costs in the United States were over 130 billion dollars.[54] Between 1974 and 1991, medical malpractice costs increased from $900 million to over $9 billion ($4.9 billion, according to Ralph Nader)[55]—an average annual increase of 15 percent (versus an 11-percent annual increase in total healthcare expenditures over the same period).[56] But the concomitant explosion of medical malpractice costs would suggest that despite the many litigation-driven "improvements" in obstetrics, ten times more negligence occurs now than twenty years ago.

To cope with malpractice, obstetricians have exchanged twelve or more years of training for a strategy which fixates on the worst possible outcome and relies on the most extreme, interventionist (but not necessarily effective) treatment option to prevent it. One consequence is that the rate of cesarean births in this country has increased multifold from 4.5 percent in 1965 to a high of 24.1 percent in 1986.[57, 58] (While the average cesarean delivery rate in this nation hovers between 20 and 25 percent, sixteen hospitals had cesarean rates of over 45 percent in 1989 and 1990, according to the Public Citizen's Health Research Group.[59] America's highest cesarean delivery rate during this period occurred in a Louisiana hospital with a frequency of cesarean birth of 57.5 percent.) Yet despite an avalanche of medicolegal litigation, the rates of cerebral palsy (i.e., brain damage) and prematurity have remained unchanged for decades. A. Russell Localio of Pennsylvania State University noted a paradoxical relationship between malpractice claims and cesarean delivery rates.[60] Mr. Localio found that in New York state, cesarean delivery rates were lowest in counties with low rates of malpractice claims and higher in counties with higher rates of litigation, leading to inevitable questions as to whether obstetricians are influenced more by legal fears than they are by medical ones. After all, wouldn't it make more sense for higher cesarean delivery rates to be associated with lower rates of malpractice claims?

The explosion of malpractice claims over the past twenty-four years hasn't necessarily improved the health of Americans. Rather, it has spurred on the surge of claims to greater heights. One Chicago law firm, for example, recently informed its clients: "We are pleased to announce that we obtained for our client the largest verdict ever for an arm amputation—$7.8 million."[61] Peter W. Huber, himself a lawyer and outspoken critic of nonsensical liability claims, notes:

> Verdicts speak to the public at large, too, and people tend to believe what the courts say, especially when they say it with large amounts of money. The casual follower of jury verdicts might easily conclude that most pelvic disease is caused by IUD's and tampons, most lung disease by workplace dust and building asbestos, most road injuries by defects in car design, and most miscarriages, birth defects, and cancers by medicinal drugs, pollution, or obstetrical incompetence. But they aren't.[62]

One study found that more than 80 percent of malpractice claims filed against New York physicians were without merit.[63] But even when no malpractice has occurred, the obstetrician can ill-afford going to court to

93

prove it. The disruption to his/her practice that a three- to six-week malpractice trial would bring makes defending him/herself an undue **94** hardship, especially for his or her patients. Indeed, it's easier and less disruptive to quickly settle out of court. Besides, most out-of-court settlements are paid by the doctor's malpractice insurance company, not the doctor him/herself. Personal injury lawyers exploit this issue, often mounting what is essentially a shake-down. In fact, a considerable number of personal injury lawyers earn handsome incomes from out-of-court settlements—sometimes going long stretches without actually setting foot in court.

The Data Bank

The National Practitioner Data Bank (NPDB) is a clearinghouse supposedly designed to ensure that clinics, hospitals, and health insurance companies know the malpractice history of a given physician. The Data Bank was established under the Health Care Quality Improvement Act of 1986. Under the terms of the act, state licensing boards, hospitals, and other health care entities are required to report to the Data Bank adverse licensing and disciplinary actions taken against practitioners. Likewise, malpractice insurers must report all payments made on behalf of individual practitioners. According to Ralph Nader, "it helps to identify bad doctors likely to commit future acts of malpractice."[64] But does it?

Review of information from the Data Bank's first four years of operation (1990–94) yields confusing results.[65] Perhaps most puzzling of all is the utter disconnection between medical mischief and malpractice payments:

Disclosable Reports (Rank)	Malpractice Payments (Rank)
1. Connecticut	1. Montana
2. Hawaii	2. Michigan
3. Massachusetts	3. West Virginia
4. Illinois	4. Wyoming
5. New York	5. Nevada
6. Minnesota	6. Pennsylvania
7. Pennsylvania	7. Kansas
8. Rhode Island	8. New York
9. North Carolina	9. Texas
10. Louisiana	10. Louisiana

Reprinted with permission of Oxford University Press from R. E. Oshel, T. Croft, J. Rodak. "The National Practitioner Data Bank: The First 4 Years." *Public Health Reports.* 110(July/August 1995)383.

If we look at states at the bottom of the list, things get even more confusing:

Disclosable Reports (Rank)	Malpractice Payments (Rank)
42. Wyoming	42. Wisconsin
43. Indiana	43. Maine
44. North Dakota	44. Minnesota
45. Nebraska	45. Massachusetts
46. Kansas	46. Connecticut
47. Montana	47. District of Columbia
48. Colorado	48. Maryland
49. Arizona	49. South Carolina
50. District of Columbia	50. Hawaii
51. Nevada	51. Alabama

Reprinted with permission of Oxford University Press from R. E. Oshel, T. Croft, J. Rodak. "The National Practitioner Data Bank: The First 4 Years." *Public Health Reports.* 110(July/August 1995)383.

With few exceptions, there's no apparent correlation between a given state's frequency of disclosable reports and malpractice payments. In some cases, the relationship is absolutely contrary to what one might reasonably expect. For example, Montana, the state with the most malpractice payments, ranked forty-seventh with regards to disclosable reports. Conversely, Connecticut had the greatest number of disclosable reports, yet ranked near the bottom (forty-sixth) when it came to malpractice payouts. Does this suggest that Connecticut's doctors are the nation's worst? Are Montanans America's most litigious citizens? There's no way to know. But what the data does show is that the relationship between medical misbehavior and malpractice payments is far from clear-cut. Contrary to Mr. Nader's assertions that the NPDB would ferret out the bad apples, the data suggests that—at least in civil court—some of our nation's worst medical offenders are escaping the consequences of their actions while others are being unduly pursued.

The NPDB requires reporting of malpractice verdicts, disciplinary suspensions, and license revocations so as to supposedly prevent bad physicians from moving from state to state to practice (i.e., to protect consumers from recidivist doctors). However, a recent study found no correlation between the prior malpractice claims of over 230 Floridian obstetricians and the technical quality of care they provided.[66] At least two other researchers were also unable to demonstrate that malpractice claims data could reliably predict future physician performance.[67, 68] Moreover, the United States Department of Health and Human Services has found that NPDB information influences credentialing committees' decisions to grant doctors hospital privileges only one percent of the time and that state medical licensing boards are not influenced at all.[69]

Examples

There are three prime examples of medicolegal meddling which deserve mention in regards to the health of American women:

BENDECTIN

Hyperemesis gravidarum is a severe, protracted, potentially life-threatening form of morning sickness. Affected patients may become severely dehydrated and experience metabolic derangements capable of compromising mother and child. Pregnant women can die from this malady. In 1956, Bendectin was approved by the Food and Drug Administration (FDA) for the treatment of hyperemesis and was used by roughly thirty million pregnant women. Yet more than twenty years after its approval, the *National Enquirer* attributed thousands of "hideous birth defects" to the use of this medication.[70] Supposed "experts" likened Bendectin to thalidomide, the notorious drug that was connected to terrible birth defects in the early 1960s. The result: millions of dollars in claims against Bendectin's manufacturer for alleged birth defects supported by so-called experts and their questionable research. Ultimately, the credentials and theories of these persons were dismissed: over thirty epidemiologic studies concluded that Bendectin didn't cause birth defects.[71] The World Health Organization, the FDA, and the March of Dimes concurred. Bendectin, one of the best-studied drugs in history, was safe for use in pregnancy after all. In court, Bendectin's manufacturers eventually prevailed, but not until after they had spent one hundred million dollars for its defense. Tired of doing battle in court, the manufacturer removed the exonerated medication from the market in 1983. Since Bendectin was pulled from the market, the Centers for Disease Control has detected no significant decrease in the incidence of birth defects.[72] However, the number of hospitalizations for hyperemesis gravidarum has doubled. Thus, it would appear that the only people to have benefited from this litigation-induced change in medical care are lawyers. "If you're suffering from morning sickness," quips one industry cynic, "go see your lawyer."[73]

THE INTRAUTERINE DEVICE

The intrauterine device (IUD) is an effective form of contraception. For   **97** certain women with conditions that contraindicate other contraceptive modalities, the IUD is the only reliable form of birth control they can use. As with all forms of birth control, patients must be properly selected. But when certain criteria are met, the IUD is a safe, effective contraceptive. Unfortunately, intrauterine devices have been painted with the same brush as the notorious Dalkon Shield, a specific type of IUD shown to cause injury to the female reproductive tract. Other IUD's weren't associated with the same risks and were eventually cleared by epidemiologic studies.

Notwithstanding, personal injury attorneys pursued the other IUD's, eventually sweeping them from the market and leaving a considerable number of women without a safe birth control method. Indeed, for many with significant medical problems, pregnancy is a more dangerous, life-threatening condition than any potential risk posed by the IUD. New versions of the IUD have crept back onto the market in recent years. But the high costs (due in part to the built-in expenses to help cover future potential litigation) may keep the IUD out of reach for some who truly need it. Moreover, the consent form that must be read and signed can be daunting and disheartening for prospective users.

SILICONE-GEL BREAST IMPLANTS

As many as two million women have received breast implants filled with silicone gel in the United States and Canada since 1962.[74, 75] Since 1982, a small number of patients with connective-tissue illnesses in conjunction with silicone breast implants have been reported. Predictably, a well-publicized onslaught of litigation against the makers of the implants has followed. Despite monetary settlements that have to date exceeded several billion dollars, at least ten published medical reports have failed to demonstrate any relationship between silicone implants and connective-tissue infirmities.[76–85]

The most recent report was conducted by Dr. Jorge Sanchez-Guerrero at Harvard University.[86] Among nearly 88,000 women who were monitored for fourteen years, Dr. Sanchez-Guerrero not only found no increased risk for connective-tissue disease, he was unable to demonstrate any increased occurrence of 41 signs or symptoms even suggestive of the malady. Moreover, the American College of Rheumatology (doctors who specialize in diseases like those supposedly caused by silicone) recently announced that it sees "compelling evidence that silicone implants expose patients to no demonstrable additional risk for connective tissue or rheumatic disease."[87] While implant litigants have been quick to point out that the Food and Drug Administration (FDA) banned silicone implants for cosmetic surgery, they seldom volunteer the fact that the FDA's action in 1992 was not prompted by concerns that the implants were harmful.[88] Rather, they were pulled from the market because manufacturers hadn't completed certain legally required studies of the implants—an altogether different issue. Indeed, the FDA agreed that silicone implants should remain available for reconstructive purposes (e.g., following disfiguring cancer surgery). To top things off, a distinguished British medical panel convened by the British Minister for Health to study the issue concluded that silicone-gel implants were no riskier than other implants. Reporting on the panel's findings, Anna Vondrak of Knight-Ridder/Tribune News Service concluded that:

> Science eventually has triumphed, but the only clear winners are a handful of plaintiffs' lawyers who have stuffed their pockets with fistfuls of dollars. The biggest losers, unfortunately, are the women who have been gulled by the plaintiffs' lawyers. Many went to great expense to have their implants removed—most often unnecessarily. Others had real but curable illnesses that went undiagnosed because they believed their lawyers' spiel that implants were to blame.[89]

Having witnessed the pillage, makers of other silicone medical products may soon stop or limit their manufacture. Pacemakers, lens implants, and artificial joints for our parents as well as dialysis tubing and ventricular shunts for our children may vanish from the market even though no credible medical evidence against silicone exists. According to Dr. Katherine Dowling at the University of Southern California School of Medicine, "Most medical class-action suits, with their often weak to non-existent standards of proof of harm, may end up costing those in need of medical devices and implants dearly."[90]

Consider the following facts, as provided by Dr. Frank H. Boehm in an editorial from *MD News of Greater Phoenix:*[91]

- 79 percent of obstetricians in the United States have been sued at least once and 25 percent have been sued at least four times.
- As of 1990, over 12 percent of obstetricians have stopped practicing obstetrics due to liability concerns and 24 percent have re-

duced the number of high-risk pregnancies for which they are providing care.

- A recent AMA-sponsored Gallup Poll of over 1,000 practicing doc-   **99**
tors found that 84 percent of physicians order extra tests to protect themselves against malpractice lawsuits. Defensive medical practices have been estimated to add fifty billion dollars to the annual cost of healthcare.

Factors which help determine whether malpractice suits are filed frequently have less to do with whether malpractice has occurred than with the personality of the physician. According to Dr. Gerald Hickson at Vanderbilt University, physicians are more likely to be sued if patients feel they're rude, if they rush visits or fail to answer questions.[92] One of Dr. Hickson's studies analyzed almost 1,000 obstetricians to discover what made patients happy with their medical care. Patients were asked how long they had to wait before seeing a doctor, how much time they spent with the doctor, whether the doctor treated them respectfully, and whether the doctor listened to their concerns and questions. Obstetricians who'd been sued the most scored the lowest in almost all of Dr. Hickson's survey questions. Moreover, patients of the most frequently sued physicians reported twice as many instances where the physicians actually shouted at them.

By contrast, physicians who'd never been sued were most likely to be seen by their patients as concerned, accessible, and willing to communicate. A study by Dr. Howard B. Beckman at the University of Rochester confirms Dr. Hickson's findings.[93] Dr. Beckman reviewed forty-five plaintiffs' depositions from settled malpractice suits between 1985 and 1987, identifying problematic doctor-patient relationship issues in 71 percent of cases.

Is every doctor who is sued a bad doctor? Dr. Stephen S. Entman, also of Vanderbilt University, studied the relationship between obstetricians with a history of malpractice claims and the quality of care they provided five to ten years after those claims.[94] Dr. Entman found no difference in the technical care provided by physicians who'd been sued and those who hadn't. According to Dr. Hickson, "These studies show that a doctor might not have done anything technically wrong but generated enough misunderstanding and anger to provoke a malpractice claim." More direct are the comments of Dr. Sidney M. Wolfe, a consumer advocate with the Public Citizen Health Research Group, who notes, "A doctor can't get away with being a technical whiz and an interpersonal jerk."[95]

Contingency Fees

100   After convincing a jury that a victim of medical malpractice deserves millions of dollars for her hardship, the lawyer skims off 33 to 50 percent. The lawyer's portion of the earnings represents his/her contingency fee. After the lawyer has taken his/her cut, the client's award is whittled further by court costs such as expert witness fees, confirmatory medical tests, legal filings, and private investigators. Indeed, a study of automobile accident cases associated with serious injury revealed that victims actually received less money when they hired lawyers to represent them.[96] Yet, whenever tort reform is proposed, attorneys predictably protest that the contingency fee arrangement must not be changed, arguing that without it the "rich and powerful" would exploit the less advantaged by forcing them to pay for their lawyers out of their own pockets.[97] Without the contingency fee arrangement, attorneys claim that the poor would lose access to the legal system. Dr. Jeffrey P. Phelan, a maternal-fetal specialist and attorney in Los Angeles, takes issue with the assertions of malpractice attorneys:

> The contingency fee arrangement is the tool with which rich and powerful plaintiffs' lawyers exploit the less advantaged. . . . [The claim] about contingency fees granting the poor access to the legal system is nothing but self-serving, self-righteous platitude. . . . All too often, plaintiffs' lawyers turn down meritorious cases likely to result in low payouts so as to be free to pursue questionable cases that hold out the chance of a big score.[98]

Exactly how much of the financial expenditures that are funneled into our medical-legal system actually lands in the pockets of victims? To answer that question, a study at Wayne State University in Detroit investigated the economic cost of the medical-legal tort system at Detroit Medical Center.[99] Ultimately, it was determined that only about 12 percent of the medical-legal expenditures at Detroit Medical Center actually went to individual alleged victims. Relatively recently, "no-fault" compensation has been proposed as a method for improving the current system. In theory, no-fault compensation has some potential benefits. Because negligence is not a criterion for obtaining payment, a considerable amount of overhead is eliminated. As a result, compensation could potentially also be available for injuries for which negligence did not occur or for which negligence could not be proved. Unfortunately, a study of Florida and Virginia obstetricians found that no-fault compensation had only a minor impact.[100] Another study of no-fault compensation in Florida found that payments to lawyers fell considerably. Unfortunately, Dr. Frank A. Sloan, the study's author, found that because of the narrow statutory definitions used in the system, many children with birth-related neurologic injuries did not qualify for coverage.[101]

Between January 1990 and June 1994, plaintiffs' attorneys in Alabama, California, and Texas contributed $17.3 million to candidates for state office, 10 times more than "Big Oil" and nearly 5,000 times more than the "Big Three" automakers contributed to candidates in those states during the same period.[102] Plaintiffs' attorneys' contributions to candidates in Alabama, California, and Texas nearly doubled what the Democratic and Republican National committees contributed to their state and local candidates, as well as the state parties in all fifty states.[103] According to Dr. Phelan, much of that money went to state legislators who vote to kill tort reform measures. He notes that other contributions helped elect or re-elect the judges who hear malpractice cases and appeals of those cases. The ethical dilemma this poses for state court judges is obvious as they raise large sums of money for their campaign funds, considerable portions of which are provided by the very plaintiffs' lawyers who argue before them in court. Nationally, trial lawyers made over forty million dollars in campaign contributions in 1994. In the opinion of legal expert Peter Huber, "Modern lawyers will quickly understand—though only slowly admit—how profit can corrupt their own endeavors, for they spend much of their time explaining how profit has corrupted everyone else's. The hunted and the hunters, it turns out, have far more in common than the hunters care to admit."[104]

Managed Care

For years, we lamented the socialization of medicine but were fairly unprepared for its commercialization. Yet "managed care" is a health insurance modality which is likely to be with us for the foreseeable future, so an examination of its potential effects on American pregnancies is warranted.

The idea behind managed care isn't new, nor is the aversion that doctors have traditionally had to it. During the mid 1800s in Kershaw County, South Carolina, for example, Dr. Simon Baruch was chastised by the county medical society for offering to provide medical care to local plantation slaves for two dollars each per year.[105] Likewise, the founders of the Western Clinic were drummed out of the Pierce County (Washington) Medical Society for accepting fifty cents per member per month from a group of lumber mill workers near Tacoma around 1900.[106] Organized medicine of the day abhorred contract medicine because physicians had to compete for contracts, thereby driving down the price of medical care.[107]

102

During the Great Depression, patients paid monthly dues to co-ops which then covered their medical bills. Likewise, the Farm Security Administration made loans to farmers during the Depression years, forming a healthcare co-op when it found that many of its farmers were unable to repay their loans due to poor health.[108] A popular magazine of the day likened the Farm Security Administration's efforts to socialized medicine. Indeed, the lack of a national healthcare program during the Depression was due in large part to the relative strength of organized medicine in persuading Congress against it, according to Dr. Thomas Rowland of the South Atlantic Association of Obstetricians and Gynecologists.[109] Resistance to contract medicine persisted well into the 1920s. In Oklahoma, for instance, Dr. Michaele Shahid was expelled from his county and state medical societies for founding the first hospital owned by what was essentially a "capitated" plan (shares went for 50 dollars).[110] On a larger scale, in 1929, at the behest of a Texas school superintendent, Baylor University Hospital agreed to provide 1,500 Texas teachers up to three weeks of hospital care for six dollars per teacher per year, a program which was the forerunner of Blue Cross.[111]

After the American Medical Association (AMA) was indicted for violation of the Sherman Antitrust Act, organized resistance to insurance coverage for physicians' expenses waned. In 1938, Dr. Sidney Garfield built a portable ten-bed hospital to render care at remote construction sites. Henry Kaiser, a contractor at the Grand Coulee Dam, arranged for Dr. Garfield to provide for the medical needs of his workers (another version of the story involves the Hoover Dam).[112, 113] In time, Kaiser extended the service to other businesses, thereby laying the groundwork for the Kaiser-Permanente health maintenance organization.

As the cost and maldistribution of physicians increased, the Committee on Cost of Medical Care was formed. Headed by Dr. R. L. Wilmer, a past president of the AMA and a former Secretary of the Interior under Herbert Hoover, the committee's report recommended the use of prepaid group practice for future healthcare in America, a proposal which the AMA branded as "socialization and communism" and as "inciting revolution."[114] But with the passage of the Taft-Hartley Act of 1947 which permitted welfare funds for workers to be partially funded by employers, businesses were allowed to pay healthcare premiums as business expenses for employees who received healthcare benefits as tax-free income.[115] Once again, the AMA objected to prepaid health plans, this time on the grounds that they were unethical and unfair to fee-for-service physicians. Taking their cue from the AMA, medical societies from across the nation excluded doctors from their ranks who participated in prepaid healthcare groups. Some states even went so far as to outlaw health plans that were not controlled by doctors. Given the AMA's historically entrenched attitude, it should come as no surprise that the organization was against the creation of Medicare in 1965.

Over time, it became apparent that health insurers were unconcerned about healthcare costs as long as employers were able to afford the premiums. Indeed, it's been estimated that each automobile which rolls off of America's assembly lines has a base cost of $1,200 to provide healthcare to the nation's autoworkers.[116] Medicare and Medicaid proved to be just as insensitive as commercial health insurers to costs as long as taxpayers were willing to shoulder the expense.[117] Moreover, its lucrative fee-for-service reimbursement system made it ripe for abuse.[118–120]

The HMO Act of 1973 gave federal monies to health maintenance organizations (HMO's) with the idea of putting Medicare and Medicaid on a managed care basis so as to cut expenses. As of 1997, nearly 40 percent of the Medicaid population were enrolled in managed care plans. Meanwhile, managed care in the private sector continued to make gains in the 1970s, '80s and '90s, moving to the forefront of current efforts to control our nation's healthcare costs. By 1998, roughly fifty-eight million Americans (22 percent of the population) were enrolled in managed care plans, with obstetricians having the highest rates of participation (91 percent) among so-called "primary care" specialists used by women.[121, 122] Currently, three of every four persons receiving healthcare benefits through their employers are on some form of managed care.[123]

What Is Managed Care?

Despite the uproar over managed care, there is no universally agreed-upon definition as to what it actually is. Thus, it's worthwhile to consider how health insurance used to work and how it has changed under managed care. Traditionally, doctors worked on a fee-for-service basis (i.e., "pay-for-what-you-get"), similar to any traditional business in America. Whatever the doctor charged is what the patient or his/her insurance company would pay. But unlike other businesses in America, physicians were immune to market forces

104

because doctors in the fee-for-service (FFS) era didn't compete against one another for customers. As more physicians moved into a given community, their fees didn't fall, nor did poor service put economic pressure on subpar doctors to go out of business the way any other inferior product would be driven from the market. In essence, physicians operating under the traditional system were a cartel whose income and political clout were protected via local medical societies on up through national organizations such as the AMA. The more services a FFS doctor rendered, the more money he/she made, his/her fees being set by what the market would bear. Patients who couldn't pay were forced to seek care elsewhere unless the doctors accepted "charity cases." Undesirable clientele could also be turned away at the discretion of the doctors.

Unlike any other business, demand for healthcare grew as the number of doctors and hospitals increased in the FFS era. In chapter 3, we saw how the immigration of neurosurgeons into Maine paradoxically produced a surge in the number of citizens "in need of" neurosurgery. (In a logical world, one would expect that the need for neurosurgery would precede the influx of neurosurgeons.) But Maine's experience was not unique in the days of FFS care. New Hampshire provides yet another example: after a new open-heart surgical unit opened in Manchester, there was a 100-percent increase in the number of open-heart procedures. Moreover, this type of surgery became more common with progressively less severe cases of heart disease. Unfortunately, there was no improvement in mortality from cardiovascular disease in the community, despite the fact that twice as much "care" was being rendered. Under the FFS system, according to Dr. Derek van Amerongen of Johns Hopkins University Medical Center, "We as physicians have been completely unaffected by the costs of treatment . . . encouraging waste and inefficiency, rewarding marginal care, and demanding no accounting for quality—regardless of the degree of mismanagement or inappropriateness."[124]

Managed care changes traditional FFS healthcare by supposedly integrating and overseeing the provision and financing of medical care, its aim allegedly being to improve the quality of care while simultaneously controlling costs.[125] Under managed care, both patient and doctor are supervised (i.e., "managed") by way of restrictions that limit a patient's choice of caregivers and medical options, and which regulates the clinical autonomy of physicians.[126] Under managed care, there are a variety of ways that patient care may be provided and an equally diverse range of reimbursement methods for doctors.

Components of Managed Care

For an excellent, more detailed review of managed care's constituent parts,   **105**
the reader is urged to read Dr. Elizabeth A. McGlynn's article on the topic
in the journal, *Women's Health Issues.*[127] For the purposes of our discussion,
the following is sufficient:

The Benefits Package. The benefits package is essentially the contract between
patient and insurer. The benefits package outlines the medical services to be
covered and sets out the conditions under which care may be accessed.[128] In
a closed network, patients will be covered by the health plan only if they seek
care from physicians who are members of the health plan's restricted network.[129] Participating doctors are usually catalogued in a "providers man-
ual" supplied by the health plan. Closed networks seem to be the most onerous type of network for both patients and physicians because they interfere
with patients' choices and doctors' independence, possibly compromising
the "patient-doctor" relationship. A point-of-service network allows patients to go outside of the plan's physician network if the patients are willing
to pay a larger share of the expenses generated.[130] Other plans may operate
on a gatekeeper system which controls access to specialists. In this model, patients select a primary care physician with whom they must initiate all medical contacts. If the patient bypasses the gatekeeper, the managed care plan
will not pay for the specialty services rendered. Due to the volume and complexity of the benefits package, there are many opportunities for confusion,
misinterpretation, and error, especially at the level of the "fine print."

Physician Reimbursement. There are a number of ways doctors are paid for
their services by health plans:

- *Fee-for-service (FFS).* As mentioned earlier, this is the "pay-for-what-
  you-get" system which health insurers are trying to undo with managed care.
- *Discounted FFS.* In exchange for ensuring that the health plan will
  send patients to a particular doctor, the doctor accepts a smaller but
  guaranteed portion of what would have been charged under the traditional FFS system.[131] The actual discount is negotiated between the
  doctor and the health plan.
- *Salaried Arrangements.* Under a salaried arrangement, the doctor is
  hired by the health plan and provides care to health plan enrollees for

a salary.[132] Kaiser-Permanente and CIGNA health plans are examples of this type of managed care known as health maintenance organizations (HMO's). Physicians under this arrangement are sometimes paid bonuses, depending on their "productivity" and/or the fiscal success of the health plan.

- *Capitation*. With capitation, the healthcare plan pays the primary care/gatekeeper physician a lump-sum fee to provide healthcare for a given patient for a prescribed period of time during which the gatekeeper pays for all contracted medical services. He or she has complete freedom as to how, when, and by whom the patient is treated. But if a particular patient requires care that costs more than the lump-sum fee, the physician must cover the costs him/herself. On the other hand, any residual funds at the end of the term are kept by the physician as profit:

Earnings (negotiated fee paid up-front to doctor)
− Expenses (referrals, treatments, etc.)

= Profit (or deficit)

Needless to say, the managed care landscape is littered with ethical potholes. Under such a system, the goal is to control the delivery of unnecessary or ineffective care that may diminish profits. From the health plans' perspective, the best care will be less care, and that is where the trouble begins.

According to Dr. Marc A. Rodwin of Indiana University,

Managed care organizations structure the delivery of medical care to limit patients' choices and control. They restrict choices by implicitly excluding medical services through management decisions that limit the resources available to physicians (such as reducing budgets for equipment), by imposing rules and incentives that encourage physicians to practice more frugally and thus not consider or recommend certain medical options, and by explicitly excluding certain medical services from the benefits package. . . . Implicit methods of restricting services—by resource management or rules and incentives—hide from patients their limited choices.[133]

There is perhaps no other enterprise where profits grow when less service is provided. This topsy-turvy relationship is enforced through health plan decisions which limit the resources available to doctors and by giving them incentive to practice more economically. After a capitated managed care plan

is instituted in a community, office visits and specialty referrals have been observed to dwindle almost immediately and hospital occupancy rates sometimes decrease dramatically. Indeed, it's been estimated that if capitation was   **107**
instituted nationwide, there would be a surplus of medical specialists as a
consequence of decreased utilization. Thus, the individual doctor faced with
a system less dependent upon his/her services will either be forced to play
the managed care game or find him/herself outside the system.

The Problem

Healthcare in America is expensive. The costs of maternal and infant care,
for example, easily exceed thirty billion dollars annually, and someone has
to pay for it. But someone is also profiting. Exactly who the beneficiary is
depends in part on whether the healthcare being provided is based on FFS
or managed care. A necessary backdrop to this discussion is the definition
of what sufficient, appropriate healthcare is and whose definition of it
should apply (see What Kind of Healthcare Should Be Covered, later in
this chapter).

In an ideal world, healthcare would be universally available and there
would be an unlimited supply of money to support it. Moreover, all services—from the mundane to the esoteric or experimental—would be covered
and, at the same time, care would never be rendered simply to line caregivers' pockets. But in reality, funding for healthcare is not infinite. As a result, choices must be made regarding its delivery which produce winners and
losers in the healthcare game.

It's a generally held notion that physicians are supposed to act on behalf
on their patients, using their discretion and expertise for the exclusive benefit of their patients; in other words, doctors have a fiduciary relationship with
their patients. But because managed care creates financial incentives for doctors to control costs, it could be argued that this type of health insurance creates a conflict with a physician's fiduciary responsibility. Lost in the argument, however, is the fact that FFS arrangements also promote conflicts of
interest for the doctor, albeit of a different nature. Remember, under managed care, less care saves money while under FFS, more care makes money.
With the former, patients are supposedly being denied necessary care (to the
financial benefit of insurance plans), whereas in the latter, unnecessary care
is being foisted on patients (to the financial gain of physicians). The truth of
the matter is that all financial incentives are problematic when it comes to
healthcare.

108   A recent study by Dr. Scott B. Ransom in Detroit illustrates the phenomenon: During a six-month period at Hutzel Hospital and the Henry Ford
Health System, obstetricians monitored in the study performed 15 percent
more surgery under FFS reimbursement than they did during a six-month
period under a capitated managed care system.[134] Moreover, Dr. Ransom
found that the increase in surgery was entirely due to elective (i.e., non-es-
sential) procedures. The frequency of essential surgeries was no different
under the two different types of health insurance. According to Ransom,
"Until now, I had been operating under the admittedly naïve assumption
that the practice of medicine is motivated almost solely by benevolence and
concern for people."[135] Another example of the influence of money on doctors comes from Montana, where in 1997 the Federal Trade Commission ordered a hospital and a physician trade group in Billings to "cease and desist"
from collusive behavior which, according to Elliott Blair Smith of *USA
Today*, developed into a price-fixing cartel which may have cost Montana
consumers millions of dollars.[136]

  Throughout modern times, organized medicine in America has opposed
attempts (or perceived attempts) to control doctors' income, impugning the
ethics or motivations of their nemeses much the same way that managed care
organizations are being attacked today. Physicians' efforts to combat managed care have been joined by the popular press which laments almost
weekly the problems with this type of health insurance. But do we really
want to return to a system of healthcare whereby physicians could do essentially as they pleased and be remunerated without concern for the appropriateness of their management, with no attention to patient outcomes or quality of care? Is managed care really worse than a system where doctors could
turn away poor, minority, and/or Medicaid patients? After all, it was the ex-
cesses of the fee-for-service era which gave impetus to the growth of managed care in the first place. Moreover, as Dr. Robert St. Peter of Mathemat-
ica Policy Research points out, it's important to remember that many of the
same physicians who practiced under the old fee-for-service system are now
working under managed care.[137] Also worth remembering is the fact that
during the "good old days" of fee-for-service medicine, Congress had to
enact the Pregnancy Discrimination Act of 1978 to force employers to provide maternity health services in the same manner that coverage for other
medical services was provided.[138]

  On the other hand, health insurance companies that utilize managed care
have realized sizable cost savings and profits. While there are a number of
things which health insurers can do with their new-found earnings, one op-

tion would include passing the savings on to customers, thereby making health insurance coverage more accessible. Based on recent history, however, it appears that insurers don't always do this, even when the law mandates it. **109** For example, a United States District Judge recently ruled that Blue Cross of Ohio improperly pocketed secret discounts that it obtained from hospitals instead of passing them on to its enrollees.[139] In Florida, Humana, Inc., paid $6.25 million in 1994 to settle allegations that it overcharged 37,000 enrollees by not passing along discounts as high as 89 percent.[140] Moreover, in New York, 500 doctors filed a class-action lawsuit in 1998 against a local HMO for non-payment of more than $140 million in fees. According to Dr. Hugh R. K. Barber, editor of *The Female Patient*, "HMO's claim that the only way to make a profit in healthcare is to cut services, perpetrate fraud, or both. . . . Therefore, if high profits and individualized care are mutually exclusive—as industry executives claim—it follows that any hospital, clinic or HMO reporting high profits deserves careful scrutiny."[141] Dr. Charles Phillips, a California physician, has taken matters into his own hands against what he calls "mangled care" with a web site (http://www.balancedcare.net) where he shares the text of a book in progress and invites readers to provide input. His book details stories of patient disasters spawned by denial of treatment, improper diagnoses and mistimed hospital discharges, all of which allegedly occurred in order to save money.

Discussions about managed care are often portrayed as battles between good and evil when the truth is that the fight is largely about money and control. Neither doctors nor managed care plans are above reproach in this controversy. At the heart of managed care is the goal of reducing costs by controlling access to medical services. From patients' perspectives, it appears that they are being denied necessary care, a notion which doctors who yearn for the days of FFS are more than happy to encourage. Indeed, a study conducted in 1994 found that 38 percent of managed care enrollees were concerned that their health plans might deny them medical treatment at some point in order to save money,[142] while in that same year, Massachusetts doctors sued an HMO plan for allegedly cutting corners on patient care.[143] In the hit movie *As Good As It Gets*, audiences actually applauded when one of the movie's characters complained about dealing with HMO's. Nevertheless, Dr. Mark R. Chassin, Chairman of Mount Sinai School of Medicine's Department of Health Policy and Mount Sinai Hospital's Senior Vice President for Clinical Quality, estimates that at least 20 percent of what doctors do represents overuse and could be eliminated without adverse effects.[144]

From the doctors' point of view, managed care has brought with it unwelcome intrusion and interference. They are frustrated with the flood of external control into their clinical practices. The gatekeeper arrangement of some managed care plans has created a burdensome authorization system which reduces efficiency. A maze of utilization reviews, claims administration, pre-admission certifications, benefits eligibility determinations, global service fees, and diagnosis-related groups have increased doctors' administrative load and their cost of practice. To make matters worse, each insurer has its own unique contracting and authorization procedures, thereby increasing the complexity of the process. As one who has been there, it's almost as if the system is designed to discourage all but the most strident or persistent requests for referrals, hospitalizations, or treatments. Indeed, given the complexity and time-consuming nature of some authorization processes, many doctors likely think twice before pursuing more extensive diagnostic or therapeutic regimens for some patients.

Competition in the health plan marketplace has resulted in economic incentives for purchasers of health services (i.e., employers) to change health plans frequently. As a result, continuity of care is sometimes disrupted as patients switch from one provider network to another. Doctors are also being paid less per patient under many forms of managed care, but they're making up for it by seeing more patients. To accommodate a larger patient load, office visits are shortened, a trend which is unsettling for patients. Thus, managed care as it frequently functions has the potential to erode the doctor-patient relationship by way of productivity pressures, economic disincentives against continuity of care, and potential conflicts of interest between doctors and patients.

In the face of patients' and doctors' healthcare concerns, many managed care plans are reaping sizable profits and rewarding their leaders with lavish economic rewards. The burdensome administrative components of managed care plans are also seen as unwieldy and inefficient drains on health plans' economic resources, resources which some say would be better spent on improving benefits packages for enrollees. Indeed, according to Marianne M. Jennings of the Lincoln Center for Applied Ethics at Arizona State University, 24 percent of all healthcare dollars are spent on administrative costs.[145] According to Dr. Jeffrey P. Phelan, editor of *OB/GYN Management*, obstetricians' earnings fell more than 5 percent in 1995, yet the average number of patients seen per week rose from 94 to 104.[146] At the same time, health insurance premiums are increasing roughly 3 percent annually, prompting Dr. Phelan to ask in a recent editorial, "Where is all the money going?"

One explanation is that costly new technologies and drugs are to blame, as is the rapidly growing number of elderly people who require healthcare. But this is only part of the explanation. As mentioned earlier, the reality is **111** that a significant share of the nation's healthcare expenditures are not spent on actual patient care, but for administrative costs and industry profits. Indeed, the Health Care Financing Administration (HCFA) predicts that HMO profits will account for even more of the growth in spending than they presently do because HMO's can no longer shrink their margins to gain market share.[147] But it's not illegal to reap large profits if it is done within the constraints of applicable regulations, and a health plan may use its money as it sees fit. While this may seem unfair to the patient who has been denied a medical service, there is currently little that can be done about it. On the other hand, many managed care plans may be in serious financial trouble. For example, California's Senate Insurance Committee was recently advised that 50 to 90 percent of that state's medical providers are experiencing financial difficulties.[148] Likewise, Weiss Ratings, the insurance rating agency, found that more than 35 percent of the 510 HMO's it monitors are in bad fiscal condition, thereby placing the healthcare of millions of patients—including pregnant ones—in potential jeopardy.[149]

As mentioned in chapter 3, some managed care plans may also be contributing to the phenomenon of perinatal deregionalization. In their search for cost savings, managed care plans will sometimes develop their own perinatal or neonatal centers which compete with established regional centers, thereby diluting the clinical experience and expertise in a given area. While a managed care plan may be able to run its own neonatal intensive care unit more economically than an established center of excellence, the data shows that it may be doing so at the cost of babies' well-being.

Quality of Care

For all the economic benefits that proponents of managed care tout, there's scant data regarding the quality of medical care provided under this system. Some in the industry feel that meaningful monitoring of quality is still years away. Meanwhile, will women with pregnancy complications be referred to appropriate levels of care or will obstetricians be forced to keep them at outpost hospitals while trying their luck at treating them and saving money at the same time? Will managed care devise a way to promote quality and not just economic expedience, or will we allow personal injury attorneys to "fix" the system for us?

112   It isn't clear if quality should be defined by those who provide care or those who receive it. According to the Institute of Medicine, quality is "The extent to which health services for individuals and populations increase the likelihood of desired health outcomes and are consistent with current professional knowledge."[150] When it comes to quality, there are at least three aspects of healthcare which may be evaluated: the structure of care (e.g., the proportion of network doctors who are board certified, the ratio of doctors to enrollees, etc.), the healthcare process (e.g., the proportion of women who receive Pap smears, or the percentage of children who receive immunizations), and patient outcome assessments.[151] Thus far, quality assessment of managed care plans has emphasized the structural and process-oriented aspects of care, in part because they are easier to track. The interpersonal and outcome-oriented aspects of care have been less easy to measure. After all, accessing administrative data such as the proportion of women undergoing Pap screening is less taxing than determining if the Pap screens were properly done or if patients had their questions satisfactorily answered. As a result, most so-called quality measures have been fairly crude, focusing more on aspects of care which can be easily tabulated rather than those which must be dissected and studied. The current tools for measuring quality of care are more like inventories than they are meaningful assessments of healthcare excellence. The difference in this circumstance is like the difference between reading a grocery store's produce list and actually sampling the goods.

When managed care comes to town, what amounts to a game of "chicken" begins for local doctors. As long as they all shun the managed health plan's overtures, it is quite difficult for the plan to make inroads. But when the first few physicians sign up with the emerging network, the united front crumbles and the floodgates open to managed care. While no one wants to be the first to cave in to a managed care plan, no one wants to wait too long and risk being "locked out" of a health plan once it has contracted with a sufficient number of doctors in a given community to establish a presence in the local market. Doctors that a particular managed care plan doesn't select for participation in its network are not allowed to provide care for patients covered by that health plan. As a result, doctors who have been locked out can lose a sizable share of their clientele virtually overnight as patients are forced to switch to doctors who are within the plan.

What is it that makes one group of physicians more attractive to a managed care plan than a competing group? It frequently has little to do with quality. Managed care plans are often attracted to physicians with a large patient base, especially if the health plan is trying to penetrate a new market. Other times, managed care plans are drawn to more efficient groups that are **113** more capable of controlling their costs. Thus, managed care companies tend to recruit larger, more cost-conscious practices at the expense of smaller ones and make them even larger. Those who are unable or unwilling to vie for participation in managed care plans may find themselves out of business. Larger groups of physicians who resist the managed care juggernaut may also encounter trouble. For example, the physician-run Marshfield (Wisconsin) Clinic was sued on antitrust grounds by Blue Cross and Blue Shield of Wisconsin when the clinic refused to accept a capitation agreement. Managed care plans are driven by price to a much greater extent than they are by quality. Low-cost doctors are rewarded irrespective of the quality of care they provide. Thus, many managed care plans aren't able or motivated to identify, much less sanction, bad physicians.

According to *OB/GYN Management,* managed care plans' reliance on capitation is likely to increase. Indeed, the publication's editors anticipate that "Obstetricians and gynecologists will have to boost patient volume and reduce encounter time to maintain income."[152] As a result, American mothers can expect to see the conveyor-belt style of prenatal care already prevalent with many obstetricians intensified. There will be even less time for the very aspect of prenatal care that may be most valuable—the interpersonal relationship between the mother and her prenatal care provider. Moreover, as doctors become increasingly focused on efficiency, they'll be less able to stay current on topics in their specialty. As Dr. Greg McGrew admits in the *Journal of Practice Building Strategies,* an advertising circular published quarterly by the Evergreen Group in Irvine, California, "I no longer have time to sit down in my office with a cup of coffee and catch up on my professional journals . . . but I'll pay that price for a healthy practice that is equipped to compete in today's healthcare war zone."[153]

ERISA

Although the doctor practicing within a managed care system will need to limit patients' access to the medical system, he/she will still need to practice defensive medicine because managed care offers no special protection from malpractice claims. In fact, it may actually increase medicolegal liability for physicians: many health insurance companies shoulder almost no responsibility for bad outcomes because a law by the name of the Employment

114

Retirement Income Security Act (ERISA) of 1974 shields some managed care plans from litigation. As established by Congress, ERISA preempts potential claims against some managed care plans that would ordinarily be governed by traditional tort law. Under ERISA, a mother claiming she was improperly denied a benefit—an ultrasound, for example—is entitled to recover only the cost of the ultrasound. Should she experience an adverse outcome stemming from the managed care company's behavior, her obstetrician would be the only viable target of a liability claim.

A real-life example of this phenomenon comes from Alabama where United Health Care and Blue Cross were sued for the death of an unborn child: The mother of a "high-risk" pregnancy was advised by her obstetrician to be hospitalized for the duration of her pregnancy so as to more closely monitor her fetus.[154] However, hospitalization was deemed unnecessary by United Health Care, a utilization review organization for Blue Cross (utilization review organizations advise health plans about the medical necessity of what their network doctors are prescribing for enrollees). Instead of hospitalization, United Health Care authorized ten hours of home nursing per day. Unfortunately, the fetus succumbed while the nurse was off duty. Because the insurance plan was an ERISA plan, the court found that ERISA shielded Blue Cross from the suit.

By design, ERISA hinders the regulation of managed care at the state level. This phenomenon is a result of Congress which, late in the process of debating ERISA, chose to override state laws pertaining to pension plans, including healthcare. But while ERISA established uniform standards for pensions, it failed to do so for health plans. Thus, ERISA doesn't require health plans to offer specific benefits or to meet standards regarding contracting with physicians, payment rates, or even patient care. To make matters worse, most courts have held that ERISA prohibits states from requiring ERISA plans to disclose information regarding how the plans are administered or how they decide claims.

Managed Care and Medicaid

Medicaid was created in 1965 as part of the legislation which created Medicare.[155] As mentioned earlier, virtually all participating physicians of the day were reimbursed on a fee-for-service basis. In 1982, Arizona, which until that time had no Medicaid program, enrolled all of its eligible citizens in managed care plans, becoming the first state to be granted the necessary exemptions from the Department of Health and Human Ser-

vices for a statewide Medicaid program based solely on contracts with
managed care plans.[156] Since that time, Medicaid has increasingly moved
into managed care; as mentioned earlier, almost 40 percent of Medicaid   **115**
patients—largely low-income women and children—are presently enrolled
in managed care plans.

Because pregnancy is one way to qualify for Medicaid coverage, Medicaid
plays a large role in financing maternity care, covering nearly 40 percent of
births in this country.[157] Indeed, Medicaid is the leading financer of births in
the United States, thereby making prenatal care a prioritized issue for Medicaid managed care. Pregnant women on Medicaid—poor and disproportionately minority—were traditionally shunted to overloaded inner-city clinics and hospitals, in large part because they were not welcomed elsewhere.
Indeed, Tennessee's managed care Medicaid program ran into problems
when that state's private Blue Cross plan told doctors in its provider network
that they would have to accept managed care Medicaid ("Tenn-Care") patients in order to remain in the provider network.[158, 159] Rather than accept
the so-called "cram-down" rule, however, nearly half of Tennessee's 7,000
Blue Cross doctors dropped out of the plan, re-enrolling only after it became
evident that their practices were not economically viable without Blue Cross
patients.

As private insurers have increasingly turned to managed care, however,
Medicaid managed care plans have become increasingly attractive to some
healthcare providers. In fact, many Medicaid plans now pay doctors as much
or more than private managed care companies, and they frequently pay
faster.[160] Suddenly, private hospitals and physicians are scrambling for low-
income pregnant women—now among the most lucrative patients in the
healthcare business. So aggressively has the industry been courting these
once-spurned patients that some use inducements to attract them. Low-income mothers-to-be are now invited to baby showers, given baby clothes,
monogrammed blankets, or car seats.[161] In the past, private hospitals had no
interest in low-income pregnant women. Prenatal care for the poor, if it was
available at all in some areas, was found only in county healthcare facilities.
But as private hospitals and physicians felt the squeeze of managed care, and
as many Medicaid programs boosted their reimbursement rates, low-income
pregnant women were suddenly an attractive market. Some private hospitals
now go so far as to send workers into poor neighborhoods in search of pregnant women to be enlisted into their maternity programs.[162] As a further incentive, private hospitals can qualify for even more federal funds for indi-
gent-care services (thereby receiving what can amount to millions of dollars

of additional income) if a sufficient number of Medicaid mothers are enrolled.[163] Meanwhile, around the nation, county hospitals traditionally run on Medicaid dollars have seen their patient populations dwindle as attractively decorated private hospitals and private doctors skim off patients that they previously would have refused to accept.

116

But is the new attitude towards low-income pregnant women the product of altruism or changing economic tides? In fact, the pursuit of Medicaid pregnancies may represent an example of cherry picking, whereby the most lucrative patients are sought by the players in the healthcare game. One doesn't see these same hospitals and caregivers clamoring for terminal cancer or AIDS patients precisely because they are less profitable. To this end, the comments of Dr. Fred Gober, an Atlanta obstetrician, merit consideration: "If Medicaid pregnancies were to become less financially appealing to healthcare providers, all the hospitals that are fighting for Medicaid will bail out in two seconds. Patients will be left in the lurch."[164]

Managed Care's Performance

Dr. Robert H. Miller of the University of California in San Francisco compared the healthcare utilization, expenditures, quality of care, and patient satisfaction in managed care (HMO) against indemnity (i.e., traditional health insurance) plans from 1980 through 1993.[165] Dr. Miller found that compared to indemnity plans, HMO's had 26 to 37 percent fewer hospitalizations, 1 to 20 percent shorter hospital stays, at least as many office visits to the doctor per enrollee, less frequent use of expensive procedures and tests, greater use of preventive services, comparable results regarding outcomes (fourteen of seventeen observations showed either better or equivalent quality-of-care results), somewhat lower enrollee satisfaction with their services (seven of eight observations showed that fewer enrollees were as satisfied with their care), and higher satisfaction with costs (one observation revealed 13 percent lower expenditures for HMO enrollees while another report showed at least 11 percent lower expenditures). While managed care horror stories are in vogue in the popular press, there is at least some evidence that women's healthcare hasn't fared so badly under managed care. In 1977, for example, only 57 percent of new health insurance policies (most of which were based on the old fee-for-service system) offered some form of maternity benefits, prompting Congress to enact the Pregnancy Discrimination Act of 1978, mentioned earlier.[166–168] According to Dr. Elizabeth A. McGlynn of the RAND Health Program in Santa Monica, California, a routine gynecologic exam is covered in 99 percent of managed care plans, compared to 49 percent of indemnity plans.[169] Moreover, coverage for some form of contraception is offered in 93 percent of managed care plans versus only 51 percent of indemnity plans.[170]

117

The Medicaid Competition Demonstrations were conducted to compare a managed care version of Medicaid against traditional Medicaid programs.[171-173] Of the three categories of care relevant to women (preventive services, prenatal care/pregnancy outcomes, and care for acute problems), all of the differences that were found favored the managed care plans. With regard to prenatal care, there were few differences between managed care and traditional Medicaid, and no differences in outcome (i.e., pregnancy outcomes were no worse with managed care). In other studies, greater use of preventive services (including Pap smears, breast exams, and mammography) was found to occur in HMO's, compared to FFS plans. Managed care has also spurred the drive towards practice guidelines—something that many independent-minded physicians detest—to help doctors update and standardize their clinical practices by incorporating the latest research into their clinical management of patients. Managed care is also slowly moving towards quality measurement of healthcare delivery and towards providing physicians with feedback on variations in their practices which may be impacting patient outcomes. It also emphasizes primary care and incentivizes the coordination of care and communication among caregivers. Thus, in contrast to how it has been portrayed, managed care actually possesses some features which may be beneficial, particularly with regards to women's healthcare, even though the evidence doesn't suggest that pregnancy outcomes are any better under managed care than they were with other type of reimbursement.

What Kind of Healthcare Should Be Covered?

Besides the issues of money and control, the managed care debate could be framed in terms of what constitutes appropriate healthcare. While few would argue that garden-variety health services (i.e., broken bones, appendicitis, etc.) shouldn't be covered by whatever type of healthcare plan we utilize, there's much less agreement on just about everything else. Are our healthcare dollars better spent providing diagnostic and therapeutic services for a disease like breast cancer, which affects roughly one in ten American women, or should we use those same dollars to fund experimental treatments for less frequent but very expensive kinds of other diseases? And what impetus

118   should there be for managed care plans to cover new, unproven diagnostic or therapeutic tools? Unfortunately, most Americans—and a large number of physicians—confuse new or different regimens as automatically better than standard-fare medicine, especially when the disease in question is serious or potentially deadly. But when healthcare dollars are thrown after untested or ultimately ineffective nostrums, time, money, and emotional capital are squandered. It's one thing for a managed care plan to obstruct access to those forms of healthcare that have been shown to be effective; this type of behavior should be exposed and punished. It's an entirely different issue, however, when managed care plans balk at covering an emerging regimen without sufficient, convincing data supporting its effectiveness. More care isn't always better care, and new treatments don't necessarily promote healthier lives; that's just the way it is. But new treatments are almost always more expensive than traditional care and therefore have the potential to force changes in how health services are provided.

If you were the director of a health plan with a fixed operating budget, would you choose to pay for an unproven AIDS treatment for a single tragic patient, or would you use your funds to pay for a thousand Pap smears? In the days of unlimited healthcare dollars, such issues would be moot, but in today's world, there are few absolute solutions to our problems. Instead, healthcare problems and their solutions are best viewed in terms of tradeoffs, as Dr. Thomas H. Sowell of the Hoover Institute at Stanford University would suggest.[174] Is a managed care plan's refusal to cover home uterine activity monitoring or a subcutaneous terbutaline pump device evidence of a greedy corporate decision to save money, or is it a rational decision based on the unimpressive medical evidence that either of these two "breakthroughs" actually help pregnant women? While a health plan's decision to deny such treatments to pregnant women provides excellent fodder for the evening news, it may nevertheless be the correct medical decision.

On the other hand, managed care's attempts to cut back on the delivery of certain healthcare services should be subject to the same scrutiny as those who seek to add new, untested medical regimens. Unfortunately, the issue of managed care has been politicized by all involved. Indeed, much of the current anti-managed care rhetoric is generated by physicians angry over the changes befalling their profession and by politicians looking for an issue to exploit, in the opinion of Dolores Mitchell, Executive Director of the Massachusetts Healthcare Purchaser Group.[175] Ultimately, this is a battle between freewheeling FFS medicine and the hucksterism of the medical-industrial complex it promotes on one extreme, and the overbearing, profit-driven megasystems which flourish on the backs of patients on the other. It is a battle loaded with politics, power, and money. As is typically the case, careers will rise and fall as this drama plays itself out. Left in the middle will be our pregnant women.

A prime example of what happens when medicine and politics collide may be found in the issue of so-called "drive-through deliveries": Contemporary postpartum care has its roots in the charitable maternity hospitals of the seventeenth and eighteenth centuries where new mothers underwent a strict twenty-eight-day regimen of "lying-in."[176] By World War II, most deliveries were occurring in hospitals where new mothers stayed for roughly a week. Up through this era, almost every instance where shorter hospital stays were encouraged, the driving force was the economic and logistical needs of the hospitals themselves.[177] But the further shortening of postpartum hospital stays which began in the 1970s was largely the result of mothers' own demands as they took a more active role in their healthcare.[178] More recently, many contemporary obstetrics textbooks suggested that the typical postpartum stay following a vaginal delivery was two to three days and that the usual post-cesarean convalescence was four to five. With the rise of managed care, however, hospital stays following vaginal births fell to twenty-four hours or less and uncomplicated cesarean patients were sometimes dismissed in two days, thereby giving rise to the "drive-through delivery" moniker. Thus, the problem was described as one of unduly short postpartum hospital stays and the poor maternal and infant outcomes that critics were certain would result, and managed care was seen as the culprit because foreshortened hospital stays of healthy mothers were pushed by managed care plans in order to save money.

Armed with little more than presumptions about what constituted the appropriate lengths of postpartum stays, opponents of drive-through deliveries went to work. By the end of 1996, thirty-two states and the United States Congress had passed legislation which mandated how long mothers and newborns were to be hospitalized, generally two and four days following vaginal and cesarean deliveries, respectively.[179] Problem solved? It depends on one's perspective. While ensuring that new mothers and their babies aren't rushed out of the hospital after delivery is certainly a well-intentioned idea, there's no medical evidence whatsoever which suggests what the optimal length of hospitalization following childbirth should be. Indeed, almost thirty studies have been published, the large majority of which found no adverse effects of early postpartum dismissal (i.e., discharge less than two days after a vaginal birth and three days or less after a cesarean). A study of early post-cesarean dismissal which I co-authored found that over half of the postoperative complications which occurred didn't develop until the fifth postoperative day or later (i.e., well after mothers would have gone home, even under the new provisions).[180] To be fair, an independent review of published evidence regarding early dismissal found virtually all of the studies to have flaws. Nevertheless, the reviewer, Dr. Kenneth E. Grullon of the University of California in San Francisco, concluded that early postpartum discharge was probably safe for properly selected patients.[181]

The amount of intensive, individualized care which occurs in the first few postpartum days in a hospital is generally much less than proponents of longer postpartum stays might imagine. What exactly occurs during the post-delivery hospitalization of healthy mothers? In theory, they're receiving ample rest and education. But due to the lower "acuity" of patient care that is required, postpartum wards are sometimes staffed with a single registered nurse; the rest are merely assistants. Moreover, most busy medical centers aren't terribly restful or private places, especially if a mother must share a semi-private room with another new mother. The postpartum recovery period lasts six weeks; whether or not a patient is given extra time in the hospital after childbirth cannot overcome the conditions which may exist in the woman's home environment.

Clearly, a new mother could use help around the home after delivery, but is this to be the responsibility of the hospital, doctor, or health plan for otherwise healthy women? Traditionally, the "helper" role was played by friends and family, but with an ever-mobile society, the breakdown of traditional social and family ties, and the rise of single parenthood, our customary support systems have become more tenuous. Will the problems of contemporary convalescence become yet another social issue which we will repair via medicalization? Perhaps we as a society will choose to do so, but what will be the tradeoffs? And where is the data to support it? Unencumbered by data (or rather, in spite of the data), opponents of drive-through deliveries "solved" the problem first by politicizing it, then by legislating it out of existence. Armed with anecdotes and good intentions, these activists secured longer postpartum stays without taking steps to ensure that busy hospitals would (or could) provide sufficient nursing personnel to cover the logjams which inevitably arise from longer hospital stays. In the words of a letter sent by the entire maternity nursing staff to the director of a major southwestern U.S. hospital:

There are many days patients wait long hours in the waiting room for beds to become available . . . or for an available nurse to assume their care. . . . We see many of our colleagues becoming burned-out from the constant **121** and unrelenting stress. The turnover rate within our unit is astronomical. The pool of experienced nurses is continually being diluted and morale is at rock-bottom. Some quit before completing orientation. Others leave for less demanding jobs, imposing less professional risk. Those with experience are too busy picking up the slack and assuming care of the more difficult patients to find time to mentor the newer staff.[182]

Strength in Numbers

The recent spate of mergers among health insurance companies has occurred for a number of reasons. But the primary reason has nothing to do with the well-being of patients. First and foremost, mergers are occurring so as to increase the profitability of the insurance companies involved. Unfortunately, it is unlikely that any newfound profits will result in better insurance coverage or lower premiums for their enrollees.

Among doctors, there is growing interest in the formation of a nationwide union to combat the growing power and influence that health insurance companies wield over them. Ostensibly, this tactic is being undertaken by physicians on behalf of their patients so as to regain control of the medical decision-making process. But another motive which drives the pro-union movement is the desire to combat insurer-driven cuts in physician reimbursements by establishing a unionized physician fee scale.

What We Can Do about It: Step Four

1. Altered Expectations

Despite contemporary trends that encourage greater participation of the patient in her own health maintenance, we continue to foster the notion that pregnancy is not a self-sustaining system. By promoting a culture that depends on a medicalized system of prenatal care, a tacit agreement has been reached between society and physicians that simply cannot be met. Bad outcomes occur and always will. Despite our many technologic advances, sometimes there is nothing we can offer the mother. As we have seen, the effectiveness of a considerable number of things that we do for complicated pregnancies is not supported by scientific data. By cornering the prenatal care market, however, obstetricians have set a trap for themselves with the undue high faith and expectations invested in them by their patients. Indeed, it is these expectations that become the malpractice attorney's refrain when bad outcomes occur. Nevertheless, the medicalized culture of American prenatal care contains within it traditions and norms which patients have come to demand and by which obstetricians are measured. Based upon the mediocre pregnancy outcomes that American prenatal care provides and the expense that such care generates, one must conclude that the quality of American prenatal care is overrated. While this fact may be disquieting to pregnant women in this country, it is nevertheless true. Having been told for so long that the American medical system is the finest in the world, most assume that our prenatal care system is similarly blessed. The reality is that, given the state of the present system, we must reconsider just how much benefit prenatal care American-style actually provides.

2. Changes in the Nature of Prenatal Care Itself

After devoting an entire book to its inadequacies, it would be illogical to advocate greater access to American prenatal care as it presently exists. As we have seen, strategies seeking to improve access to prenatal care have not improved prenatal care utilization or pregnancy outcomes. Moreover, intensified prenatal programs have failed to impact targeted high-risk groups while unbridled technologic advances have increased expenses without improving outcomes. What is needed is a prenatal care system that is simpler, less medicalized, and more widely distributed throughout our communities so as to encourage American women's participation in it.

EMPHASIZE QUALITY OVER QUANTITY

Bigger Is Not Better. In other healthcare specialties, sick patients may tolerate interpersonal lapses if they believe that their doctors will "cure" them. However, healthy mothers ambivalent about being pregnant may be less likely to abstain from unhealthy activities or to comply with inconvenient prenatal regimens if the advice to do so comes from a caregiver perceived as indifferent or with whom they have little in common. The generally superior levels of satisfaction noted among nurse-midwives' patients are a reflection of the strong relationship between mother and caregiver. We must ensure that such relationships are fostered instead of streamlined.

Few human service-oriented businesses handle large volumes of customers well, especially when the services provided are complex. Therefore, it should be anticipated that managed-care systems designed to abbreviate prenatal visits that are already remarkably short and unproductive will further harm the quality of our prenatal system. The "take a number" philosophy has no place in prenatal care. Instead of larger, busier clinics designed for efficiency, we must seek a greater number of small clinics that are more widely dispersed throughout our communities.

Fewer Prenatal Care Visits. Most prenatal visits are pointless and unrewarding for the mother. Exceedingly little time is allotted for education or meaningful interaction with the actual prenatal care provider. Indeed, mothers often spend more time with ancillary obstetrical personnel or waiting for the doctor than they do actually receiving care from him/her. In a medicalized prenatal care system based on the premise that each pregnancy is a process waiting to go awry, when disease has been ruled out, there's nothing more to talk about. Prenatal care should be based on the assumption that each low-risk pregnancy is normal until proven otherwise. Pregnancy is not disease—it should not be subjected to the same style of care that the ill must endure. Prenatal visits should be infrequent and deliberate. Ample time should be scheduled for questions and reassurance. Each visit should conform to a curriculum of maternal education designed to inform mothers about pregnancy and childbirth, foster personal health maintenance, and dissuade unhealthy behaviors. Each prenatal care visit should be conducted by the mother's actual prenatal care provider—as few ancillary personnel as possible should come between mothers and caregivers. Mothers should come away from each visit better prepared for the remainder of pregnancy. Among low-risk mothers, the requisite number of prenatal visits could likely be halved without compromising quality of care. Indeed, high-quality, low-frequency prenatal care visits that emphasize the educational and emotional aspects of maternal health would likely produce better compliance and higher levels of maternal satisfaction.

Nontraditional Hours. Traditionally, physicians' offices have operated during regular business hours, an average of four and one-half days per week and almost never on weekends. With the premise that healthcare is an important commodity, it is puzzling that supermarkets and fast-food shops keep more convenient hours than most medical clinics. In an era where many American women have jobs outside the home, scheduling working mothers' prenatal visits during business hours is certainly not in their best interests. Prenatal clinics that operate after regular business hours and on weekends would offer a variety of advantages for expectant mothers. First, nontraditional hours would reduce time conflicts between mother's jobs and prenatal visits. Second, nontraditional hours would allow fathers and other working family members to accompany mothers to their prenatal visits, thereby allowing greater family participation and support. After-hours clinics would also allow mothers greater access to transportation from working friends and family members. Lastly, after-hours clinics would allow greater access to childcare from friends and family who cannot provide it during business hours. Traditional prenatal clinics have operated for the convenience of doctors, not mothers. Nontraditional office hours would remove a significant logistical barrier, thereby improving otherwise motivated mothers' prenatal clinic attendance.

Nontraditional Locations. Historically, prenatal care has been provided by physicians in their offices. As doctors have migrated to medical office complexes in the vicinity of hospitals, they have become relatively isolated from patients. In some cases, mothers travel considerable distances to visit their obstetricians in areas sometimes unfamiliar or uninviting to them. There is nothing about prenatal care that requires it be dispensed from a medical office. To the extent that prenatal clinics are located in places that foster usage by mothers, mothers will be better served. In step with the idea that we should have a larger number of small prenatal clinics is the notion that these clinics be more accessible. Prenatal clinics should be located where mothers live—in their neighborhood community centers, malls, churches, mosques and other local institutions. As such, mothers could receive prenatal care with and from others in their locality, thereby reducing transportation and childcare concerns. Moreover, by drawing upon neighborhood resources, a greater sense of community may be fostered and local/cultural mores may be better respected. Basing prenatal care at local religious centers may also better facilitate the monitoring and support of at-risk mothers.

PHASE OUT OBSTETRICIANS FROM DIRECT PARTICIPATION IN THE PRENATAL CARE OF LOW-RISK WOMEN

Any remedy to the problem of maternity care in the United States must reverse the process of undue medicalization that has beset pregnant women. This country already has the rudiments of an effective, non-medicalized prenatal care system. Both here and abroad, certified nurse-midwives (CNM's or "nurse-midwives," not to be confused with lay midwives) have demonstrated themselves to be effective primary care providers for women of all **125** ages and socioeconomic levels. Since the 1920s when nurse-midwifery was established in the United States, nurse-midwives have been acknowledged for their role in reducing infant and maternal death. Report after report has shown that nurse-midwives produce better patient compliance and higher levels of maternal satisfaction when compared to obstetrician-based care. Midwives take less time to train, generally charge less for their services than obstetricians, and are more willing to practice in geographic areas that are eschewed by obstetricians. A growing number of doctors are recognizing that nurse-midwives may cut medical expenses and improve access to prenatal care. By giving nurse-midwives a greater role in the care of normal, low-risk pregnancies, obstetricians will be better able to direct their expertise to the minority of mothers with complicated gestations. Many European countries with better pregnancy outcomes than the United States, especially Scandinavia, give important prenatal roles to midwives:[183]

	Obstetrician*	Midwife*
Belgium	Yes	No
Denmark	2	5
Finland	No	10
France	Yes	Yes
Luxembourg	4	No
Netherlands	No	Yes
Norway	No	11
Scotland	Yes	Yes
Sweden	Yes	10
Switzerland	Yes	No
England/Wales	Yes	Yes

* Yes/No or number of visits
Reprinted by permission of Blackwell Science, Inc., from B. Blondel. "Some Characteristics of Antenatal Care in 13 European Countries." *British Journal of Obstetrics and Gynecology.* 92 (1985)565.

HISTORY OF AMERICAN MIDWIFERY

Nurse-midwifery was first introduced to the United States in the guise of the Frontier Nursing Service in Kentucky during the 1920s. The Frontier Nursing Service was instituted to provide healthcare to Appalachian families by sending public health nurses into the area on horseback. In 1929, after receiving nurse-midwifery training in Europe, Mary Breckinridge and a small number of British nurse-midwives began attending deliveries. A review of the first 1,000 deliveries performed by this group in Kentucky demonstrated no pregnancy-related maternal deaths. With the encouragement of the Children's Bureau, the first midwifery school in the United States was established in the early 1930s. A second training program was established during World War II and continues to function today, having graduated over 500 students. By the 1950s, there were seven training programs in the country as nurse-midwifery training established itself within academic settings such as Yale, Johns Hopkins, and Columbia Universities. In 1955, the American College of Nurse-Midwifery was created, becoming the American College of Nurse-Midwives (ACNM) in 1969. Presently, the ACNM serves as the professional organization for nurse-midwives in the United States. The ACNM accredits nurse-midwifery training programs and sets the standards by which nurse-midwifery is provided in America. Since the profession's inception, its acceptance and popularity have steadily increased. Over 4,000 nurse-midwives were practicing in the early 1990s. In 1992, they participated in over 175,000 deliveries in the United States.[184]

EDUCATION OF MIDWIVES

A CNM is a primary care provider for low-risk prenatal, delivery, newborn, and well-woman gynecologic care. The majority of CNM's hold masters or doctoral degrees. Indeed, among all nurses with advanced education, nurse-midwives have the largest proportion that hold doctoral degrees. Prior to entering nurse-midwifery training, the student must be a registered nurse. The designation of CNM is conferred after completing an accredited graduate program and passing a certification examination established by the American College of Nurse-Midwives Certification Counsel. Nurse-midwifery education entails one to three years beyond the requisite training to become a registered nurse. Nevertheless, the cost of training a nurse-midwife is one-quarter that of an obstetrician.

BARRIERS

Despite the willingness and demonstrated ability of nurse-midwives to serve pregnant American women, there is presently an insufficient number of nurse-midwives to meet the need. In a study funded in part by the Robert Wood Johnson Foundation, the ACNM determined that:[185]

- Nurse-midwives provide good pregnancy outcomes.
- Nurse-midwives save money compared to obstetricians.
- There is a shortage of nurse-midwives.
- Current levels of funding for nurse-midwifery are inadequate to meet present and future needs.
- Restrictions on nurse-midwifery limit the development of clinical teaching sites for students.

Nurse-midwives have demonstrated their ability to contain or reduce expenses while providing an excellent level of care. Historically, nurse-midwives have well served the healthcare needs of women and are poised to make a major contribution to the status of American prenatal care—if they are allowed. But as with other aspects of healthcare training, federal funds provide the bulk of support for nurse-midwifery education in America. If the role of nurse-midwives is to grow, considerably more support will be necessary to expand clinical teaching sites and increase faculty.

In 1972, Dr. Roger Egebert, a Special Assistant for Health Policy at the United States Department of Health, Education and Welfare lamented, "It is paradoxical that the Untied States, which does as well in training nurse-midwives as any nation in the world, lags so far behind other countries of making effective use of such highly trained and urgently needed healthcare professionals."[186] A variety of restrictive policies and regulations persist which have hampered the growth of nurse-midwifery training programs and the practice of nurse-midwifery. Indeed, many state regulations actually discourage midwives from seeking work. Edward S. Sekscenski at the U.S. Department of Health and Human Services in Rockville, Maryland, studied the relationship between state practice environments and the supply of nurse-midwives and found that a number of factors influenced the practice environment for nurse-midwives, such as:[187]

- Nurse-midwives' legal status as professionals in a given state.
- Whether or not reimbursement for their services is required.
- Whether or not nurse-midwives have authority to write prescriptions.

Other factors cited that might influence the practice environment for nurse-midwives included: acceptance as professionals by physicians (including collaboration and the extension of hospital privileges), inclusion in the terms of private health insurance policies, ability to obtain malpractice insurance, and acceptance by the public. Not surprisingly, favorable state practice environments for nurse-midwives were strongly associated in Sekscenski's study with a greater supply of certified nurse-midwives. As of 1994, thirty-one states allowed nurse-midwives limited prescriptive authority for medications such as prenatal vitamins, oral contraceptives, and antibiotics for urinary tract infections and vaginitis.[188]

128

There's nothing wrong with the technical aspects of care provided by obstetricians. However, the administration of effective prenatal care hardly requires the skills of physicians. Moreover, it isn't technical skill from which healthy, low-risk mothers generally benefit—especially first-time mothers. What low-risk mothers need most is their caregivers' time, a commodity in ever shorter supply in obstetricians' offices. Mothers need relationships with caregivers who are able to give the advice and reassurance they require during an important, frightening time in life. But, it's the uncommon obstetrician who has the time or inclination to foster such a relationship. Many of mothers' concerns aren't related to specific medical or obstetrical problems but instead center around direct or indirect manifestations of anxieties and emotional needs. Unfortunately, most obstetricians' goal is to address the objective, measurable components of the prenatal visit, then move on to the next patient. Indeed, it's the patient who's a "talker" that busy obstetricians dread. For the obstetrician, time truly is money, and the emotional, nonmedical aspects of prenatal care are impediments to an efficiently run office. While no obstetrician would deny the importance of the emotional well-being and education of his/her obstetric patients, few can spare twenty to forty minutes per patient per visit to provide it. Given the oppressive overhead that an obstetrician shoulders, he/she must maintain a steady stream of "low-maintenance" patients to stay solvent.

The cost of prenatal care is a recurring theme among policymakers. Dr. Elaine A. Gravely at the University of Texas in San Antonio conducted a study that compared the costs and outcomes of three different prenatal care models: Physician-based, nurse specialist-based, and "mixed" staffing clinics for low-risk mothers.[189] Dr. Gravely found no significant differences regarding maternal and neonatal outcomes among these three models of care. However, mothers receiving prenatal care from nurse specialists had significantly higher levels of satisfaction. The results of the study support those of other reports which found that nurse practitioners exhibited more interest, reduced the professional mystique of healthcare delivery, and conveyed more information than physicians. The nurse-based prenatal clinic was also less costly than the physician-based clinic—$7.81 and $11.18 per clinic appointment, respectively. According to Gravely, "The absence of significant differences among the three clinics . . . supports other reports that nurses prepared for a specific area of healthcare can provide quality care."[190]   **129**

The relationship between nurse-midwives and obstetricians in the United States has historically been a vertical one. Nurse-midwives generally exist in subordinate fashion relative to obstetricians, "supervised" by physicians for the entirety of their careers. While the intent of this arrangement has been to ensure that the midwife has someone to "help" her in the event that problems arise, it's also served to limit and control the activities of nurse-midwives. Clearly, nurse-midwives aren't trained to perform amniocentesis, external cephalic version, or other complex prenatal procedures. Fortunately, most pregnant women don't require these procedures—procedures that obstetricians themselves frequently refer to high-risk specialists. For healthy, low-risk mothers, the essential components of prenatal care remain constant irrespective of who's actually providing the care. Thus, nurse-midwives should have the same autonomy that obstetricians have to advise and care for mothers during low-risk pregnancies; restrictive regulations should be modified, limited prescriptive authority should be permitted, and greater acceptance as medical professionals by the obstetric establishment should be fostered. By the same token, nurse-midwives should be held to the same standard of care for low-risk patients to which obstetricians are held.

Most pregnant women experience relatively uncomplicated, low-risk pregnancies. Acknowledging that our ability to predict which woman will ultimately develop significant pregnancy complications is poor and that our ability to favorably alter significant pregnancy problems is also poor, the new model would send 80 to 90 percent of all pregnant women to a midwife-based system of prenatal care, with 70 to 80 percent overall remaining with a nurse-midwife through delivery. While the criteria for defining "high risk" will vary from one area to another, the consequence of such a prenatal care system is that nurse-midwives would care for the majority of pregnant American women; obstetricians would manage only complicated mothers. Clearly, such a system would require more nurse-midwives and fewer obstetricians. Given the relative paucity of nurse-midwives and the overabundance of obstetricians that the United States presently has, a system such as the one described would have to develop gradually over several decades.

Based upon the findings of the American College of Nurse-Midwives (ACNM) study discussed earlier, the following recommendations were put forth by the ACNM which may foster midwife-based prenatal care:[191]

- Include nurse-midwives as an integral part of healthcare reform.
- Increase support for nurse-midwifery education.

130

- Promote universal acceptance of full-scope nurse-midwifery practices.
- Monitor the need, demand for, and supply of nurse-midwives over time.
- Gradually adjust nurse-midwife/physician ratios within maternity care.

Increased use of nurse-midwives for prenatal care is an effective strategy which can help allay the burgeoning costs of prenatal care for women without compromising pregnancy outcomes. As outlined by the ACNM report, private industry and the government can take a number of steps to further this aim. Specifically, private industry can:[192]

- Offer prenatal care provided by nurse-midwives as an option in employee benefits packages.
- Support full payment for maternal services by nurse-midwives.

State and federal government can:

- Include nurse-midwives in the decision and policy-making process within the perinatal healthcare system.
- Encourage nurse-midwives to practice in medically underserved areas by way of educational loans, traineeships, and expansion of health service corps scholarships.
- Permit professional autonomy for nurse-midwives.

Nurse-midwives work in a variety of settings that include hospitals, birthing centers, health maintenance organizations, public health departments, private practices, and public clinics, frequently caring for women who cannot or will not seek care through more traditional avenues. As the emphasis for prenatal care delivery shifts from obstetricians to non-obstetricians, demand for the services of nurse-midwives will increase, as will the need to train more. To accomplish this aim, the ACNM report in part recommends:[193]

- Promotion of maternity and women's healthcare provided by nurse-midwives.
- Promotion of nurse-midwifery as a career choice among secondary school students.

- Increased government and private-sector funding of nurse-midwifery programs.
- Targeting of resources to nurse-midwifery training programs with the capacity to expand quickly to meet future needs.

OTHER IMPEDIMENTS TO THE ACCEPTANCE OF MIDWIVES
IN AMERICA

No small degree of antagonism has existed between the most philosophically entrenched midwives and obstetricians over the last few decades. Nurse-midwives are sometimes perceived as vestiges of a counterculture which long shunned more traditional approaches to medicine and obstetrics and thereby have made few inroads among those who sought to limit the scope of their practice. Viewed by many as a form of alternative healthcare, nurse-midwives have at times had a public relations problem. However, the aspect of nurse-midwifery that most impedes its acceptance by mainstream American women is the fact that nurse-midwives are, after all, nurses. A long-held tradition in America is that healthcare is meted out by physicians, with more specialized doctors having greater prestige. Operating within this mindset, receipt of prenatal care from one who is neither a specialist nor a physician involves considerable loss of stature, in some quarters. Implied in a shift from obstetricians to nurse-midwives, therefore, is a reduction in the quality of care among those who are uninformed regarding the truly high-caliber care provided by certified nurse-midwives in the United States.

In an environment where nurse-midwives care for the bulk of mothers and where they exist as peers with their physician counterparts, nurse-midwives' role will move from that of peripheral player to that of insider in the prenatal care process. In such a system, the nurse-midwife must come to be viewed not as an alternative healthcare provider but as a caregiver for the mainstream. While the exclusive focus of this book has been prenatal care, the intrapartum period (i.e., labor) would also be affected were the proposals advocated in this book to be adopted in the United States. Clearly, nurse-midwives aren't trained to perform operative procedures such as cesarean delivery, nor should they be. Even so, some mothers will require operative intervention during the labor process. In a group of 496 low-risk mothers receiving care from certified nurse-midwives, for example, 72 (14.5 percent) were transferred to obstetricians for delivery.[194] (Compared to a low-risk group of mothers receiving care from obstetricians, however, the nurse-midwife group had a cesarean delivery rate that was 50 percent lower.)[195]

Nevertheless, steps must be taken to ensure that operative delivery, when necessary, is still available to women receiving care from nurse-midwives. **132** Undoubtedly, such a system would require a professional relationship with, and ready access to, a physician. As it presently stands, the American College of Obstetricians and Gynecologists recommends that all maternity wards have the capacity to conduct cesarean delivery within thirty minutes of the time the procedure is deemed necessary. Extending a similar rule to nurse-midwives would seem reasonable. Under such an arrangement, obstetricians' medical liability may be allayed in that they would no longer have supervising responsibility for midwives or any untoward outcomes which may occur under midwives' care. Instead, the obstetrician would be a surgical consultant—not without liability—but at significantly less risk than with the present situation whereby the obstetrician is viewed as "captain of the ship."

3. Malpractice Reform Must Occur

The high cost of medical liability isn't absorbed by the physician—it is a business expense that's passed along to the mother. For example, a study conducted by David M. McIntosh of the Hudson Institute found that the cost of medical liability at an Indiana medical center during fiscal 1993 was $450 per patient—a sum that's greater in states with less tort reform than Indiana.[196]

The rudiments of malpractice reform arose from the malpractice insurance crisis of the 1970s.[197] The Indiana Malpractice Act of 1975, one of the most extensive reform efforts at the time, was that state's attempt to address a 410-percent rise in malpractice premiums, a 42-percent increase in malpractice claims and a 264-percent increase in malpractice awards.[198] This legislation capped total damages at $500,000, capped attorney contingency fees at 15 percent for awards over $100,000, limited physician liability to $100,000, instituted mandatory medical review panels and established a compensation fund for victims. The reforms have been consistently upheld by Indiana courts over the past two decades.[199] As a result, the threat of malpractice litigation as well as the cost of malpractice insurance in Indiana are a fraction of those in other states. For example, in 1993, orthopedic surgeons in Michigan paid an average annual malpractice premium of $109,000 compared to $11,000 for their Indiana counterparts.[200] In response to the accelerating malpractice premiums in the 1980s, further malpractice reforms were initiated. Although tort reform has consistently been shown to significantly reduce the frequency and amount of malpractice awards, medical malpractice reform exists in incomplete forms across the United States. While there are a variety of steps which may be taken to remedy the current malpractice problem, there are three that merit discussion:

LIMIT DAMAGE PAYMENTS

Outright limits on overall damage awards, though likely an effective way to cap award payments, will not likely be widely accepted and may actually thwart appropriate compensation for patients who've been genuinely wronged. Instead, limits on noneconomic damages would seem a proper substitute. Such a mechanism would be especially effective at reducing awards in states where non-economic awards compromise an undue proportion of damage awards. In one report, damage caps lowered awards by over 20 percent.[201] However, damage limits should not be our goal in and of itself. There is nothing inherently good or bad about damage caps: a low cap isn't necessarily onerous and a high limit isn't necessarily frivolous. What matters is the balance of trade-offs one gets when a cap is set at a particular level. Extremely low caps, for example, might not be sufficiently punitive for a given offender and may simply allow him/her to build the cost of malpractice into his/her operating budget. While it could be argued that lower award limits might reduce the cost of medical care, there is little evidence that doctors lower their fees in response to malpractice reform measures such as damage caps. On the other hand, absent or extremely high caps have the potential to spur on frivolous malpractice claims and may also intimidate some innocent practitioners into settling out of court for smaller sums (i.e., within the payment limits of their malpractice insurance) rather than risk losing everything at the hands of a runaway jury.

Malpractice reform should not be undertaken merely to provide relief for physicians. Although "malpractice concerns" are frequently cited as the reason why some OB/GYN's retire from the obstetric portion of their practices, the truth is that it is infrequently the only or even the most important one. Quite often, OB/GYN's who eliminate obstetrics from their practices do so because their gynecology practices have become sufficiently lucrative to support them without having to tolerate the rigors of delivering babies. Other times, older physicians' health problems force them to give up the demands of obstetrics. Few retire before they can afford to, however. To the extent that they invoke malpractice concerns as reasons for their retirement, they provide ammunition for malpractice crusaders, but they infrequently are telling the whole story.

134

Malpractice reform should be undertaken because our current system costs each of us both financially and medically. It costs us financially because the money for litigation ultimately comes out of our pockets. It costs us medically because of the pain and risk we shoulder when we are subjected to the unnecessary testing and intervention which defense-minded doctors demand. Limitless awards for non-economic injury have not improved America's pregnancy outcomes, nor have they reduced the amount of malpractice which actually occurs. That pain and suffering can be quantified, let alone compensated, is a notion which could only be encouraged by someone with a stake in the compensation, such as lawyers. As is usually the case, both sides of the malpractice debate cite concerns for the patient as their motivation. The reality, however, is that doctors don't want to acknowledge, let alone pay for, their blunders, and lawyers don't want the gravy train derailed.

Thus, the task becomes one of balancing opposing interests under the guise of justice. A wide range of options exists. One would calculate non-monetary damage awards as a multiple of the economic award. For example, pain and suffering awards would be—depending on the multiplier which is selected—double, triple, a hundred times, etc., the size of the actual monetary award. A second option would establish a fixed cap (e.g., 500,000, one million, etc.) for pain and suffering. A third would incorporate the first two options whereby the higher dollar value of the two would apply. Alternatively, the lower of the two caps could be utilized.

LIMIT ATTORNEYS' CONTINGENCY FEES

That an attorney should claim one-third or more of a damage award for him/herself is insupportable. The costs of litigation should come from the attorney's recovery, not from the client's award. Limiting attorneys' share of damage awards will also disincline them from pursuing frivolous malpractice cases. President Clinton offered very limited fee caps, proposing a limit of 33 percent of damage awards—essentially what many attorneys already charge their clients.[202] The available data suggests that 33-percent caps on attorneys' fees will not reduce overall costs. But contingency caps in the range of 15 percent, as provided by tort reform legislation in Indiana, would.[203] When the system rewards a malpractice victim's attorney as much or more than his client, the real victimization occurs. If plaintiffs' attorneys care about their clients as much as they purport, they should have no objection to a change that puts victims' interests first.

ELIMINATE JOINT AND SEVERAL LIABILITY

Joint and several liability is a legal principle whereby all members of a **135** healthcare team may be held responsible by the plaintiff in a medical malpractice suit irrespective of their role or level of involvement. The ultimate aim is to increase the likelihood that one of those named in a suit will have the economic resources to furnish a sufficiently large damage payment. Thus, many plaintiffs will frequently sue the hospital where the alleged malpractice occurred because hospitals tend to carry large liability insurance policies. Damage awards should be assigned on the basis of responsibility, not the ability to pay. Forcing the negligent party to pay is just and proper. Assigning damage awards by any measure other than responsibility only serves attorneys' economic interests and does little to further justice. Moreover, it does nothing to curtail genuine malpractice.

4. Acknowledge That Malpractice Occurs

Another aspect of malpractice deserves mention. Among prenatal care providers, there exists a relatively wide range of talent and commitment. As we've seen, the selection and education process is competitive and difficult: doctors completing their training have invested considerable amounts of money and effort. Disciplinary boards, generally composed of physicians, are hesitant to expel peers from a profession for which so much is sacrificed to achieve. Moreover, most physicians are uncomfortable with the duty of reporting inept or impaired peers. This isn't to say that obstetricians and others are unaware of incompetent or unethical counterparts: one study, for example, found that over half of surveyed malpractice plaintiffs noted that health professionals (again, other than the patients' doctors) suggested the commission of medical malpractice.[204] Dr. Gerald B. Hickson at Vanderbilt University also analyzed factors that prompted families to file malpractice claims following adverse pregnancy outcomes. Dr. Hickson found that the most frequently reported reason families filed claims was that they had been influenced by someone outside of the immediate family.[205] In more than half of the cases the influential person was a member of the medical profession. According to Ralph Nader, "Of 600,000 practicing physicians in 1992, only 300 were disciplined—not even necessarily revoked licenses—just disciplined, reprimanded, suspended license for incompetence, recklessness or criminal behavior."[206] Mr. Nader goes on to say, "There are tens of thousands of doctors—probably five to ten percent of all doctors—who are drug addicts or otherwise incapacitated to practice medicine. That means 30,000 to 60,000 incompetent doctors."

136   Extrapolating data from their 1990 report, a group from the Harvard School of Public Health testified before Congress in 1993 that an estimated 80,000 people nationwide die annually in hospitals due to medical malpractice.[207] The authors noted, "The problem is not one of too many claims being filed, but one of too few claims being filed by victims of medical malpractice against doctors and hospitals." As long ago as 1964, research revealed that 20 percent of patients admitted to the hospital suffered injury at the hands of their caregivers and that 20 percent of these injuries were serious or fatal.[208] Almost twenty years later, researchers found nearly identical statistics. Moreover, autopsy studies have shown high rates of missed diagnoses that resulted in death.[209-211] In another study on the topic of medical mishaps, it was demonstrated that an average of 1.7 errors per day occurred with each patient in an intensive care unit, 29 percent of which had the potential for serious or fatal injury.[212] Interestingly, patients in the intensive care study received an average of 178 medical "activities" each day. Thus, the 1.7 error rate corresponds to a proficiency level of 99 percent on the part of caregivers.[213] But is a 1-percent failure rate an acceptable standard? It isn't in other industries. Even if we accepted a 99.9-percent proficiency rate, for example, we'd have two unsafe landings per day at O'Hare International Airport in Chicago as well as 16,000 lost pieces of mail and 32,000 checks deducted from the wrong bank accounts hourly.[214]

Hospital care has been compared to the airline industry, another complex, risky industry. Both involve carefully chosen, highly trained personnel who perform a wide range of complicated tasks in potentially life-threatening situations. But that's where the similarities end. Airline travel is a generally safe endeavor, the product of concerted efforts through the years to minimize mistakes. The airline industry has taken great pains to optimize system designs, to standardize procedures, and to institutionalize safety. Indeed, two independent government agencies (the Federal Aviation Administration and the National Transportation Safety Board) have federally mandated responsibilities regarding safety standards.[215] In addition, a confidential reporting system for safety infractions, the Air Safety Reporting System, exists in recognition of the fact that in the past, pilots seldom reported errors if they led to disciplinary action. By comparison, accident prevention hasn't enjoyed the same level of concern in the medical profession. Instead, lawyers are left to police medical error, scavenging for cases most likely to produce large pay-offs to the exclusion of less lucrative but equally deserving victims.

Does malpractice occur? Every day. And a medical establishment that ignores or downplays its extent is only slightly less nefarious than a legal establishment that masquerades as the vehicle for raising medical standards. The relatively small number of medical blunders that are pursued in court, the nonsensical but potentially lucrative cases that lawyers do pursue, and the nationwide disconnection between disclosable incidents and malpractice awards should raise concerns about whether lawyers are pursuing the right doctors in court. Only one medical specialty—anesthesiology—has made error reduction a top priority among its practitioners.[216] And by doing so, anesthesiologists have made impressive progress in reducing bad patient outcomes. Through the incorporation of fail-safe systems and by actually training to avoid errors, the mortality rate from anesthesia has gone from one death in 10,000 to 20,000 patients to less than one in 200,000.[217]

There remain a small number of obstetricians in practice who shouldn't be—who they are is often no secret among their peers. While this is likely true in all professions, its existence among those to whom we entrust our lives is especially worrisome. A sterling academic record doesn't assure medical competence or surgical skill. There's no good correlation between one's academic record and one's clinical abilities. Good grades indicate that a person tests well—it provides no assurance that the caregiver will be compassionate or conscientious. Clearly, most obstetricians are capable and their judgment is appropriate, but a perfect résumé does not guarantee that one is above reproach. For obstetricians, more than 85 percent of payments are incurred by only 6 percent of their peers.[218] Therefore, standards of conduct must be more rigidly defined and enforced, avenues for reporting impaired or inept practitioners must be broadened and penalties—especially license revocation—must be applied more vigorously. In view of the pending oversupply of obstetricians, there will be even less reason for allowing serious or repeat offenders to continue practicing. In exchange for genuine malpractice tort reform, we in obstetrics must do our part to ensure that those in our specialty who shouldn't practice, don't practice.

5. Change the Nature of the Business

Much of the social change which has occurred in this nation has been, on one level or another, economically driven. Likewise, our longstanding healthcare problems have finally received widespread attention because they've been perceived as an economic problem by a sufficient number of policymakers to warrant action. Within this context, the managed care

138 model of prenatal care may be seen as part of the problem as well as part of the solution. As we have seen, managed care as it regards prenatal care possesses a number of drawbacks:

- The shorter visits spawned by managed care short-change pregnant women, reduce the opportunity for education, and create dissatisfaction.
- Deregionalization of prenatal/neonatal resources is sometimes fostered, thereby potentially compromising outcomes.

On the other hand, managed prenatal care has some good points:

- Premature assimilation of unproven technologies is less common.
- Superfluous components of prenatal care may eventually be eliminated.

There are two steps that should be taken to help remedy the situation:

- The present fee arrangement should be revised.
- Cognition should be reimbursed as generously as intervention is.

REVISED FEE ARRANGEMENT

Under the present system of managed care, doctors must limit their per-patient expenditures. In a prenatal practice catering to low-risk mothers, early signs and symptoms of pregnancy complications may be downplayed if subtle or infrequent, especially if they mean referral to expensive specialists. Under a revised system, specialists would be capitated while generalists would receive fee-for-service, with one proviso: the diagnostic and therapeutic regimens utilized would need to be supported by quality, peer-reviewed research. General prenatal care providers would be freed from the economic constraints of specialty referrals and transfer of complicated patients would be facilitated. After all, primary care services account for a much smaller portion of our nation's healthcare budget than do specialty healthcare services. In addition to being less expensive than high-tech specialty care, primary care is also much less likely to be over-utilized. Therefore, capitating primary healthcare services is considerably less likely to produce real cost savings. Cost containment should become the domain of specialists (i.e., those who care for patients that generate the disproportionate share of perinatal and neonatal expenses). Specialists, suddenly with an economic stake in the outcomes of pregnancies, would have the job of ensuring that pregnant women are referred before their conditions (e.g., preterm labor) are too far advanced, when possible. To do so, guidelines regarding maternal referrals—based on objective research and developed and endorsed by participating generalists and specialists—would be used to minimize mismatches between pregnancy-related conditions and levels of care. A side effect of the revised system would be the elimination of "gatekeepers," as some health plans are already doing. Some plans now view gatekeeping physicians as unnecessary sources of expense and increasingly as targets of legal claims arising from allegations of flawed referrals to specialists, according to Dr. Todd Sagin in *Healthcare Leadership Review*.[219]

COGNITION VS. INTERVENTION

For too long we've undervalued the utility of intellectually based aspects of healthcare, instead favoring intervention over cognition. Surgical procedures are more handsomely reimbursed than are consultation or patient education. In a system that economically rewards intervention, interventive procedures will flourish, irrespective of their necessity or utility. Clearly, surgical expertise requires extensive training and skill—it should be compensated. However, the disparity in reimbursement between cesarean and vaginal deliveries, for example, must not be so great as to provide incentives for cesarean deliveries. Education and counseling should be remunerated at a level that is commensurate with the value they provide.

Dr. John J. Fangman analyzed the successes and failures of prematurity prevention programs at two major healthcare organizations in Minneapolis, Minnesota. Among high-risk mothers, the contributions to preterm delivery made by physician failure, system failure, and patient failure were analyzed.[220] Only physician failure (non-compliance with preterm prevention protocols, failure to refer indicated patients to education programs, lack of response to patient concerns about preterm labor symptoms, or failure to initiate treatment when indicated) were associated with statistically significant contributions to preterm delivery.

Suboptimal outcome (e.g., low birthweight, prematurity, prolonged NICU stays, etc.) attributable to deviations from established referral protocols (i.e., guidelines for referral to specialists) should be monitored.

140   Participants who persistently deviate from referral guidelines would be sanctioned by the payor. Under such a system, guidelines would need to be constructed carefully and revised regularly. Unduly rigid protocols may stifle physicians and further bureaucratize medicine. Thus, guidelines must be broad enough to permit reasonable ranges of clinical judgment and yet sufficiently firm to ensure proper levels of care for mothers.

Proper use of the system should be rewarded. As such, part of caregivers' payment should be based upon patient satisfaction and patient outcomes. Abrasive or improper medical behavior should be economically sanctioned by the payor. Conversely, excellence would be rewarded. Practitioners with recurrent adverse outcomes attributable to deviations from guidelines or ineptitude should be removed from the plan. Thus, the combination of guidelines, outcome monitoring, and physician contingency fees would allow payors to monitor and impact quality of care.

EMPLOYERS SHOULD BE CHOOSY SHOPPERS OF HEALTHCARE

Unfortunately, a single patient has little influence over her health plan. On the other hand, corporate purchasers of healthcare can exert considerable leverage in the marketplace; they are beginning to favorably influence costs and are helping to define what quality of care is. Until recently, most companies assigned responsibility for quality assessment to managed care plans themselves. Today, however, larger companies are pushing health plans to provide higher quality, more cost-effective care. After all, healthcare is a product which employers purchase for their employees. Increasingly, employers are taking more active roles in obtaining the best product they can, especially if it improves the well-being of their workers. In short, employers are seeking their money's worth. To this end, it was employers who determined that the healthcare product they were purchasing should be evaluated on the basis of quality. One result was the Healthplan Employer Data Information Set (HEDIS), a healthcare quality evaluation which contains more than seventy standardized performance measures, 20 percent of which specifically target women's health.[221] Measurement tools like HEDIS are fairly primitive, however, tending to focus on processes of healthcare delivery rather than outcomes. But they are a start. The Foundation for Accountability (FAcct) is a consortium of public and private purchasers, consumer groups, researchers, and providers seeking to create protocols which produce the best outcomes.[222] FAcct combines patient expectations with clinical and scientific data to develop methods which hold health plans accountable for optimal outcomes and to improve upon HEDIS and other inventories. Thus, large purchasers of healthcare have gone beyond legislative and tort-based remedies to improve managed care, using their considerable consumer clout to demand certain services or considerations. Within this context, individuals can play a role in improving managed care by giving feedback about their managed care experiences to their employers, by participating in their employers' healthcare shopping process, and by encouraging their employers to use assessment tools like HEDIS and FAcct when sizing-up a health plan. In addition, those companies without sufficient size should consider joining with other small companies to form coalitions of sufficient magnitude and clout so as to obtain better performances from their health plans.

141

ERISA SHOULD BE CHANGED

Dr. Laurence B. McCullough of the Center for Medical Ethics and Health Policy in Houston argues that because managed care organizations influence the behavior of fiduciary providers (e.g., physicians) with the purpose of changing their behavior, managed care organizations share moral fiduciary responsibility with doctors for patient outcomes.[223] Indeed, managed care plans exert considerable influence over physicians. Under managed care, insurers choose which physicians in a given community will participate. Given that failure to participate in a managed care plan can have devastating economic effects on an obstetrician's practice, the choice to not participate is not usually a viable one. Faced with managed care, therefore, obstetricians really have no choice but to enroll. As such, insurers must bear some medicolegal responsibility for any adverse impact upon pregnancy outcomes that managed care may produce. While the principle that the actual wrongdoer should bear medicolegal responsibility must be honored, undue economic pressure put upon obstetricians by managed care plans must be considered when poor outcomes occur—especially since obstetricians have no real alternative except to play by insurers' rules. The protection that ERISA gives some managed care plans against litigation for improper behavior is insupportable. Indeed, 70 percent of Americans favor changing federal law to allow patients to sue their health plans, according to Kevin G. Burke, a Chicago attorney.[224] There is no reason to deprive patients of consumer protections afforded them in other commercial transactions. President Clinton's plan to mandate legal accountability for managed care plans is a step in the right direction. Failing this, the least Congress could do would be to amend ERISA so as to let individual states address the problem themselves.

Two federal bills—one Democratic and one Republican—were proposed in 1997 to establish certain federal HMO standards and to amend ERISA.[225] The Democratic version, also known as the "Patients' Bill of Rights," would require independent external appeals of grievances, information disclosure, a ban on physician gag clauses, a "prudent layperson" standard for emergency services, and liability reform. The Republican bill would not repeal the ERISA liability exclusions but would instead provide for non-binding external review and limit civil penalties for failing to provide recommended services in a timely fashion. Insurance industry lobbyists spent over three million dollars to convince the public and Congress that health insurance reform would lead to double-digit increases in healthcare premiums and ultimately more uninsured Americans, according to Wayne J. Guglielmo, senior editor for Medical Economics.[226] Indeed, one must take into consideration the unintended consequences of meddling—however well-intended—into such a large industry. Yet according to Guglielmo, a study by Coopers and Lybrand estimated that giving policyholders the right to sue their HMO's would boost their healthcare premiums by only twenty-seven cents per member per month. Likewise, the Congressional Budget Office estimated that ERISA reform would increase premiums by roughly 1.2 percent, and by 4 percent for all reform provisions taken together.[227] Clearly, repealing the ERISA preemptions would open a whole new arena for trial lawyers by providing a new deep-pocket defendant for exploitation. Repeal of ERISA preemptions would also mean an increase in some health plans' vulnerability to liability claims. But the increased vulnerability would be a relative one: health plans formerly protected by ERISA would suddenly find themselves at equal—but not greater—risk for liability as those which have never been shielded by ERISA. Even so, we shouldn't get our hopes too high over repeal of ERISA protections. According to Bill Frist, a thoracic surgeon and U.S. Senator from Tennessee, even if all quality problems could be resolved, it wouldn't benefit 70 percent of employers and nearly nine of ten Medicare beneficiaries.[228] Instead, Frist advocates the creation of the Agency for Healthcare Quality to coordinate the government's quality improvement efforts, to improve access to healthcare in underserved areas, facilitate assessment of new technology and a host of other efforts to improve the quality of healthcare in the United States.

DO NOT ALLOW MANAGED CARE PLANS TO DEREGIONALIZE
PERINATAL CARE

Deregionalization can cost babies their lives. Managed care plans should
be legally prohibited from developing perinatal/neonatal units within established regions.

Patient (Customer) Education/Questions to Ask

The language of most insurance contracts can be impenetrable. Yet, there are
certain things one should strive to learn about her health plan. Unfortunately, Americans spend, on average, less than one hour per year reviewing
their health insurance contracts, only to be surprised when they discover that
a particular service isn't covered. Review the benefit packages of your contract personally or with a company representative during "open enrollment"
windows. If possible, have your employer do the same. Remember, health
insurance is a product for sale—a smart employer should try to get the most
for his/her money. According to Karen Cheney of *Money Magazine*, you
should ask questions. What are the out-of-pocket charges? How large is the
deductible? Is the plan operating on a closed system? Is your present healthcare provider a member of the plan? If you already are enrolled in a managed
care plan, find out how your doctor gets paid.[229] You should be aware if your
doctor has an incentive to limit your access to care.[230] Many plans, however,
have "gag clauses" which prevent their contracted doctors from discussing
how they are compensated.[231] If your physician can't or won't tell you, get
a copy of the health plan's contract from your employer. Find out how qualified your primary care doctor (i.e., "gatekeeper") is for specialized procedures. One managed care plan based in California, for example, required its
general practitioners to perform a host of complex procedures (e.g., tra-
cheostomies, resetting of dislocated shoulders) for which some may not have
had expertise.[232] Ask your primary care physician directly how many times
he/she has done the procedure he/she is proposing to do on you. If he/she
performs the procedure infrequently, ask for a referral to a more experienced
doctor. Get a second opinion. Many plans will cover the costs of these.[233] If
you believe you're being denied necessary care, get a second opinion as soon
as possible. Even if you must pay for a second opinion yourself, it could lend
support should you file a grievance against your health plan.[234]

5. The Chicken or the Egg?

Imagine for a moment that our nation's maternity system is perfect, outshining even those of Japan and Sweden. In this scenario, high-quality prenatal care is widespread and every pregnant woman receives early, ample attention. Even so, a considerable portion of our maternity woes would likely persist. Having spent the majority of this book disparaging the roles of doctors, lawyers, and insurance companies in America's prenatal derby, it must also be acknowledged that no matter how excellent our system becomes, its impact will stop at the front doors of our nation's mothers. For some, pregnancy will end tragically no matter how splendid their prenatal care is while others will do well without any prenatal care at all. The essential ingredient resides with the mother herself. And like so much in obstetrics, that ingredient is not well understood. Even so, each mother brings certain traits to her pregnancy which merit closer scrutiny.

Marital Status

Illegitimacy has never been the cultural norm in any society.[1] Since 1960, however, the average age of marriage has steadily risen, causing the interval between sexual maturity and marriage to lengthen, thereby allowing a greater window of opportunity for out-of-wedlock pregnancies.[2] While unwed pregnancy has been widely discussed with regards to its effect on American society, the dialogue has ignored its more immediate effect on the pregnancy itself. Yet for each maternal age group, unmarried status increases the risk for low-birthweight babies:[3]

Low-Birthweight Infants in Arizona—1995

Mother's Age (yrs)	Married (%)	Unmarried (%)
Under 15	—	7.6
15–17	7.2	9.0
18–19	7.1	7.5
20–24	5.2	7.5
25–29	5.8	8.0
30–34	5.6	9.9
35–39	7.5	12.4
40–44	9.1	16.8
45+	15.2	—
Total	5.9	8.3

Reprinted with permission of the Arizona Department of Health Services, from C. K. Mrela. *Arizona Health Status and Vital Statistics, 1995* (Phoenix: Arizona Department of Health Services, 1996).

A host of social and economic factors contribute to increased pregnancy risks for unmarried mothers. According to Dr. David Popenoe of Rutgers University in New Brunswick, New Jersey, there are three problems with single-parent families:[4]

First, they increase poverty. Poverty and single parenthood frequently overlap as contributors to poor pregnancy outcomes. Eighty percent of children born to unwed teenage high school dropouts live in poverty, versus 8 percent of children born to high school graduates who marry and delay childbearing until age twenty.

Second, single-parent families decrease the social and emotional well-being of children. Third, they generate additional social problems. Girls from single-parent families are more likely to initiate sexual activity at an early age, are more likely to be sexually promiscuous, are more likely to be unwed teen mothers themselves, and to have failed marriages, essentially setting the stage for suboptimal pregnancy outcomes.

In Arizona, marital status showed the largest change of all pregnancy-related parameters monitored during the 1980s. Single mothers here were 64 percent more prevalent in 1989 than in 1980, but so were the consequences: by decade's end, single motherhood was also represented among a larger share of low-birthweight babies, a trend which continued in Arizona until 1994.[5] In step with Arizona's experience, MetroHealth Medical Center in Cleveland noted (over an eighteen-year period) an increase in the incidence of preterm and low-birthweight babies as the proportion of unwed mothers increased.[6] Nineteen ninety-four represented the tenth (and fortunately the last) consecutive year of large increases in non-marital childbearing nation-wide: between 1960 and 1990, America's percentage of out-of-wedlock births skyrocketed from 5 percent to 30 percent of all births.[7] Despite the media's assertions to the contrary, however, most American children still live in two-parent families.[8] According to the U.S. Census Bureau in 1994, 72 percent of all American children lived with both parents.[9] Moreover, the "unstable family" is not America's problem alone. The same problem has be-fallen Denmark, Sweden, and Germany, all nations which have lower pre-maturity and infant mortality rates than America.[10] Since 1960, the divorce rates for France and the Netherlands (both with better pregnancy outcomes than ours) have tripled and quadrupled, respectively.[11] In Canada, divorces increased fivefold, and in Britain, sixfold.[12] Over this same period, births to unmarried women in America rose by a factor of six.[13] In Canada and Britain (both with lower prematurity and infant mortality rates than ours), the ille-gitimacy rates rival America's.[14] Thus, there is no single contributor to our prematurity problem which is clear-cut or easy to understand. For example, Dr. Abbey B. Berenson at the University of Texas in Galveston, Texas, found that physical abuse of unmarried Black or white pregnant women was more common than among their married counterparts.[15] While physical abuse is always concerning, it's particularly troublesome during pregnancy in light of the association between battering and low-birthweight babies.[16] Another study found that women who were physically abused multiple times were three times more likely to have been divorced than were women who had not been abused. In step with Dr. Berenson's findings, P. J. A. Hillard noted that battered pregnant women are more likely to be divorced or separated than are those with no history of abuse.

Researchers studied the influence of marital status on pregnancy outcome on a large scale several decades ago: In 1970, for example, the British Birth Survey evaluated the pregnancy outcomes of married, divorced, and never-married mothers, noting a significant reduction in birthweight among preg-nancies in the divorced group.[17] To test the relationship between the erosion of family structure and low birthweight, a study of roughly 15,000 women was conducted by Dr. Lisa J. McIntosh at Wayne State University in De-troit.[18] Dr. McIntosh's findings demonstrated that married mothers fared better than single mothers. More importantly, however, the risks for subop-timal pregnancy outcome for women with broken marriages were consis-tently as high or higher than for never-married mothers, a fact that takes on even more significance in light of a national divorce rate that nearly tripled between 1960 and 1990. In addition, mothers in broken marriages were three times more likely to consume alcohol than were married women, three times more likely to use tobacco, six times more likely to use cocaine, and six times more likely to use heroin. Among white women delivering their first **147** babies, the proportion which is illegitimate rises as maternal IQ falls.[19] Moreover, low IQ among white women is related to low birthweight even when socioeconomic status and maternal age are taken into account.[20] Thus, a complex system of interplay and a baffling array of chicken-or-the-egg relationships stymie easy explanations of our low birthweight problem.

Teenagers

Adolescent pregnancies deserve mention in any discussion of adverse pregnancy outcome; roughly one million teenage pregnancies occur each year in the United States, resulting in half a million births to teenage girls.[21] In 1996, over 11,000 babies were born to mothers under age fifteen, according to national records.[22] Pregnancy and birth rates among American teenagers are higher than in most developed nations:[23] 10 percent of girls aged fifteen to nineteen years become pregnant in this country annually.[24] (Three of ten out-of-wedlock deliveries occur in women under twenty years of age.)[25] This phenomenon is of particular concern since teenage mothers are at increased risk for having low-birthweight babies, premature deliveries, and infants who die during the first twelve months of life.[26, 27] Moreover, 20 percent of teens who conceive will be pregnant again within twelve months, and 50 percent deliver again within thirty-two months of their first child.[28]

Dr. M. L. Blankson of the University of Alabama studied women who as teenagers delivered first and second babies, finding that adolescent mothers visited prenatal clinics earlier in gestation and made more prenatal visits with the first pregnancy than with the second.[29] Preterm delivery rates rose from 15 percent in the first to 19 percent in the second gestation (i.e., roughly twice the national average). Thus, it appears that young mothers are less likely to seek care, especially with subsequent pregnancies, thereby establishing personal healthcare patterns that are fraught with risk.

While many factors likely contribute to suboptimal pregnancy outcome among teenage mothers, it appears that adolescence itself may pose a sizable risk. Compared to mothers between the ages of fifteen and nineteen, the rate of low-birthweight babies is roughly 50 percent higher among mothers less than fifteen years of age.[30] To determine whether young maternal age possesses intrinsic risk for adverse pregnancy outcome, Alison

148 M. Fraser at the University of Utah conducted an analysis of over 134,000 young Utah women. Utah women were selected for study since mothers in this state are predominately white and married, generally receive adequate prenatal care, and usually have healthy lifestyles, thereby minimizing other factors that also impact pregnancy outcome.[31] Ms. Fraser found that among white, married mothers with education levels appropriate for their ages who received adequate prenatal care, those aged thirteen to seventeen years had a significantly greater risk than mothers aged eighteen to twenty-four years for premature delivery and low-birthweight babies. Ms. Fraser concluded, "A younger age conferred an increased risk of adverse pregnancy outcomes that was independent of important confounding sociodemographic factors."

Precocious sexual activity may also be a risk factor for poor pregnancy outcome. A study conducted by Arizona State University surveyed the sexual behavior of over 2,000 Arizona women aged eighteen to twenty-two years. The findings were alarming:[32]

- 22 percent admitted that before they were eighteen they had voluntary sex with someone they'd just met.
- 40 percent had sex on the first date.
- 6 percent exchanged sex for drugs or alcohol.
- Nearly one-third had contracted a sexually transmitted disease by age eighteen.

Moreover, the Arizona State University study found that 46 percent of those surveyed who had sex before age sixteen became pregnant by age eighteen.

In 1991, America's teenage birth rate peaked at 62.1 per 1,000 females, falling to 56.9 per 1,000 females in 1995.[33] According to the CDC, teen pregnancy rates between 1992 and 1995 were down in every state which reports the data.[34] While the decrease is a step in the right direction, it is a very small one. For example, America's teen pregnancy rate remains roughly twice that of England or Canada and about nine times as high as that of Japan or the Netherlands.[35] It also remains somewhat of a mystery as to why the decrease is occurring. Indeed, as late as 1995, most of the sexual abstinence programs were not even in operation.[36] In addition, an Institute of Medicine study in 1995 found that among 200 programs which addressed unintended pregnancies, only 23 had undergone close scrutiny, and of these, only 13 were deemed even moderately effective.[37] One possible explanation may be found in an Urban Institute study which found a 12-percent increase in the use of contraception among girls and women who started having sex in the 1990s, compared to those in the 1980s.[38]

Invisible Fathers

As more and more punitive scenarios for unwed teenage mothers are considered in Congress, paternal responsibility is largely ignored in spite of the fact that three-quarters of girls who have sex before the age of fourteen say that they were coerced, according to Ellen Goodman of the Boston Globe.[39] Moreover, Ms. Goodman relates that:

- 400 teenagers are impregnated every day by men over age twenty.
- 30 percent of fifteen-year-old mothers have sex partners who are at least six years their senior.

A recent report by the Alan Guttmacher Institute noted that men ages twenty and older are responsible for half of the babies born to girls between age fifteen to seventeen.[40] Equally disturbing is a California report claiming that adults fathered over half of the babies born to girls aged eleven to fifteen years.[41] Indeed, the California study found that among eleven- to fifteen-year-old mothers, only one in ten had sexual relations with classmates. Worse yet are the findings of a Chicago study which noted that 61 percent of teenage mothers had been abused, frequently by the fathers of their babies.[42]

Unmarried teen pregnancies represent the tip of a psychosocial iceberg. In keeping with this notion, Dr. Michael D. Benson surveyed almost 1,000 junior high schoolers in Chicago, finding a significant association between early sexual intercourse in this group and suicidal ideation.[43] According to Elayne Bennett, founder of Best Friends, an abstinence program for girls, most young girls' first sexual encounters are involuntary.[44] Yet another report (of 535 young women in Washington state) found that two-thirds who became pregnant as adolescents had been sexually abused. Specifically, 55 percent had been molested and 44 percent had been actually raped.[45] These data ought to give pause to contraceptive strategies predicated on distribution of condoms to adolescent girls.

Eighty years ago, adult fathers contributed to nine out of ten births to teenage girls.[46] Although this number has steadily fallen, adult fathers have always accounted for at least half of teenage births.[47–51] Adult males involved with teenage girls are responsible for higher rates of pregnancy, sexually transmitted diseases, and marriage than teenage fathers.[52] Adult males who **150** father children with teenage girls are also more likely to smoke, to have the lowest grade-point averages while in school, and often are paired with the very youngest of mothers.[53, 54] Compared with girls whose ages are within one year of their partners' ages, those with age differences in excess of three and a half years are more likely to be of low socioeconomic status, to have behavior problems in school, to drop out of school, to smoke or use illicit drugs, and to become sexually active at an early age.[55] In fact, it has been suggested that this profile fits a pattern of antisocial behavior, thereby creating an unhealthy milieu to which pregnancy is added and from which the risk of poor pregnancy outcome is increased.[56] A study by Don Taylor of the CDC reviewed data from over 27,000 adolescent mothers in California.[57] Taylor found that adult fathers were responsible for roughly one out of every two teen pregnancies. On average, these men were nearly six and half years older than the mothers. Teenage girls in the survey who had children by adult fathers were more likely to be on Medicaid and to receive Aid to Families with Dependent Children than teenage mothers with partners closer to their ages, suggesting that older men are less likely to provide economic support for their teenage partners.

Taylor noted that the greatest risk factor for adult paternity was inadequacy of the father's education. Indeed, the poorer his education, the higher the risk. Taylor's findings are in step with others that have surmised that adult males who impregnate teenage girls have retarded psychosocial development which causes them to seek the company of emotional and intellectual equals.[58, 59] In a study of over 36,000 pregnancies in Washington, D.C., Dr. Feroz Ahmed at the Institute for Urban Affairs and Research found that higher levels of paternal education were associated with higher numbers of prenatal care visits.[60] Similarly, Dr. Greg Alexander found that paternal education in excess of twelve years had a protective effect against low birthweight and infant mortality.[61]

That the father is also responsible for pregnancy outcome is a notion that's infrequently discussed. Indeed, little attention is paid to the role of the woman's partner during gestation. Dr. Ruth Zambrana at the University of California in Los Angeles found that the mother's relationship with the father plays a significant role in the timing of prenatal care.[62] Dr. Zambrana observed that mothers who cohabitated with their partners initiated prenatal care significantly earlier than mothers who didn't live with the fathers. Moreover, this effect was more pronounced than that produced by social support from family or friends: one study found that 92 percent of fathers attending their partners' deliveries agreed that the most important reason for being present was to support their partners.[63]

The death of a fetus or newborn is a painful experience. But it's an excellent time to gauge fathers' levels of involvement and support. Rita J. Revak-Lutz of the University of Florida conducted a study of paternal involvement in this setting, finding that cohabiting fathers were significantly more likely to be present at birth.[64] Cohabiting fathers were also significantly more likely to hold the dead child after delivery and were more likely to return with their partners for follow-up doctor visits after delivery.[65] To the extent that the abusive or detached partner can adversely impact pregnancy outcome, the converse may also be true. Increasingly, estranged fathers are being pursued for financial support of their children, yet no comparable responsibility is demanded during pregnancy. The father, if he chooses, may shirk responsibility during the prenatal period, a circumstance that appears to be particularly true among unmarried or nonmonogamous couples.

A number of studies have also demonstrated that infants whose fathers smoke have lower birthweights than those with nonsmoking fathers. To illustrate, Dr. Fernando D. Martinez at the University of Arizona found that among nonsmoking mothers, the presence of cotinine (a metabolic byproduct of nicotine) in their newborn babies' blood correlated with the number of cigarettes smoked daily by the fathers.[66] Moreover, substance abuse by the mother's partner appears to increase the risk for substance abuse by the mother herself. For example, one study noted that 88 percent of abused women's assailants were heavy consumers of alcohol.[67]

Socioeconomic Status

Low socioeconomic status increases the risk of suboptimal pregnancy outcome, especially with regards to prematurity. However, most purported associations between socioeconomic status and prematurity aren't clear-cut because socioeconomic status encompasses a broad range of demographic features, each one of which may contribute independently to prematurity.

As a result, differentiating the sheep from the wool can be vexing when it comes to socioeconomic status and pregnancy outcomes. For example, the Arizona Department of Health Services found that when pregnant women of low socioeconomic status were compared to those of higher socioeconomic status, the lower socioeconomic group tended to have less education, to be unmarried, and to smoke or drink.[68] Women of low-socioeconomic-status were also more likely to receive no prenatal care than their high-socioeconomic-status counterparts despite being eligible for state-funded prenatal care. Study after study has demonstrated increases in infant mortality rates as social class decreases. But in Sweden, where no social differences exist regarding access to healthcare, prematurity is an infrequent event compared to its frequency among other nations.[69] Social class in that nation plays only a minor role as a risk factor for infant death. Moreover, Swedish housing conditions are generally good, income differences are narrower than in many other developed countries, and genuine poverty is uncommon. Rather than class differences, much of the infant mortality that does exist in Sweden has been attributed to smoking, teenage pregnancy, short interbirth intervals, non-compliance with medical advice, or delays in seeking medical care—characteristics most prevalent among those with low socioeconomic status in America.[70–72]

To address the effect of socioeconomic status alone, Dr. Beatrice Nold at the University of California in Berkeley studied pregnancy outcomes among nearly 3,500 white military wives at eighteen U.S. military hospitals in California.[73] This group of mothers was selected in order to eliminate the influence of factors which may independently impact pregnancy outcomes. Dr. Nold found a gradient in the rates of prematurity, fetal death, and neonatal death, with the higher military ranks (i.e., higher socioeconomic status) having more favorable outcomes.

Among the many risk factors associated with low birthweight, financial status in this nation appears to be a major determinant of access to general healthcare, nutrition, and social support.[74] Moreover, economic downturns can make things even worse. In a study of prenatal care utilization and adverse pregnancy outcomes during the recession of the early 1980s, Dr. Elliot S. Fisher at the University of Washington found that the number of mothers receiving inadequate prenatal care increased in both low-income and high-income areas.[75] However, the low-birthweight rate and the prevalence of maternal anemia increased only in low-income groups. Adding to the confusion, one study found that a woman's risk of delivering a low-birthweight infant was more closely associated with the social class of her father than the social class of her husband.[76] Another study suggested that the risk for prematurity was passed from one generation to the next.[77] It remains to be determined, however, if this phenomenon represents some biologic trait which is being inherited or whether it reflects the inheritance of similar personality traits and similar economic status and the problems or benefits which derive from them.

A number of authors have noted that women delivering prematurely are **153** more commonly poor, non-white, unmarried, and also at increased risk for a variety of sexually transmitted diseases, many of which may adversely impact pregnancy by triggering premature labor. Indeed, epidemiologic observations have indirectly linked prematurity with inflammation and infection of the maternal genital tract. Thus, certain types of infections may represent an indirect biologic link between socioeconomic status and prematurity, especially prematurity which occurs as a result of preterm rupture of the protective fetal membranes.

As it turns out, the United States has the highest rate of sexually transmitted diseases of any developed country.[78] But despite the fact that five of the ten most common diseases reported to the United States Centers for Disease Control and Prevention are sexually transmitted diseases, no national system is in place to fight the epidemic. Interestingly, a Texas study found that pregnant women with documented sexually transmitted diseases (STD's) who received STD risk reduction counseling at every prenatal care visit had STD recurrence rates no different from non-pregnant women, suggesting that pregnancy did not improve maternal motivation to avoid harm in this subgroup of mothers.[79]

Dr. Paul J. Meis at the Bowman Gray School of Medicine in Winston-Salem, North Carolina, found that compared to middle-class mothers, those of lower socioeconomic status were significantly different with regards to the underlying causes of low birthweight.[80] But because current interventive strategies to prevent preterm delivery are directed at underlying causes which most frequently affect more affluent pregnant women, it's little wonder that interventive programs have had minimal success with pregnant women of lower socioeconomic status. The findings of research by Dr. Saeid B. Amini at Case Western Reserve in Cleveland, Ohio, confirm this phenomenon.[81] Dr. Amini found that between 1975 and 1992, the proportion of preterm births among private patients actually declined whereas the proportion among public (i.e., poor) patients steadily increased.

Many persons' socioeconomic status is not static. A study of income tax returns illustrated this phenomenon, finding that more than eight of ten people in the bottom 20 percent of those who filed returns in 1979 were no longer there by 1988.[82] A University of Michigan study found that between 1971 and 1978, less than half of the families remained in the same income quintile.[83] In addition, an analysis of monthly Aid to Families with Dependent Children (AFDC) data showed that 70 percent of initial episodes of welfare last two years or less.[84] The Panel Study of Income Dynamics (PSID) found that during a five-year window, 20 percent of families were poor for at least one year, but only 5 percent were poor for all five years.[85] Thus, socioeconomic status is somewhat of a moving target which confounds our understanding of its impact on pregnancy. Suffice it to say, however, that those who are at the bottom of the socioeconomic scale while pregnant are at increased risk for poor pregnancy outcomes. But pregnancy itself may also impact one's socioeconomic status. For example, according to economist Walter E. Williams at George Mason University, a married working couple who postpones pregnancy will live above the poverty line since even at minimum wage (as of 1995), they would earn 17,000 dollars, while the poverty income for a family of four is 14,763 dollars.[86] Likewise, according to Dr. Neil Gilbert at the University of California at Berkeley, three of ten AFDC-recipient mothers end up on welfare due to out-of-wedlock births.[87]

Although one can be sustained via government-sponsored subsidies of money or material goods (e.g., food, shelter) during transient hard times, there is a subgroup of welfare recipients for whom hard times are not temporary.[88] These are persons who remain at the lowest socioeconomic levels while others make their way back to self-sufficiency. Adding the factor of pregnancy to women in this setting may be counterproductive, given what we are learning about socioeconomic status and pregnancy outcome. According to Lawrence M. Mead, professor of politics at New York University, non-work is a greater problem for poor women than is out-of-wedlock birth. Dr. Mead believes that poor women have the same desire for success that others have but lack the discipline to achieve it. According to Mead, failure to get and keep jobs is more an expression of unreliability than its cause:[89]

A troubled work history . . . is seldom an accident. If non-disabled people cannot get and keep a job most of the time, the reason is usually an inability to keep commitments stretching back into school and childhood. . . . The work problem is a critical cause of the unwed pregnancy problem, but the converse is not true. . . . Once one could have argued . . . that unwed pregnancy was a cause of non-work. The belief that single mothers could not work due to childcare responsibilities was the original premise of family welfare. That view was plausible when few mothers worked and welfare families were large. It is implausible today when most mothers, single or not, are employed and most welfare mothers have only one or two children.

Women who enter the Aid to Families with Dependent Children (AFDC) program due to unwed pregnancy seem to be different from those who are pushed into the program as a result of separation/divorce or a decline in family income.[90] Compared to most who receive AFDC, unwed mothers tend to be younger and are more likely to be long-term recipients.[91] Moreover, their rates of child abuse and neglect are twice as high.[92] With the rise in illegitimacy over the last three decades coupled with welfare support of such arrangements, women have been able to bear and raise children without the financial support of men. According to Dr. Byron M. Roth, professor of psychology at Dowling College in Oakdale, New York, as the financial prospects of potential partners (and presumably the attributes that generally accompany financial stability) become less important to women, other factors tend to achieve greater importance, factors which do not necessarily promote stable families.[93] One study suggested that such men tend to be proud of their willingness to exploit women, who are frequently young girls.[94] According to Dr. Mead, out-of-wedlock pregnancy is significant less for itself than as a marker of greater problems.[95]

Thus, one is left to ask whether low socioeconomic status alone is sufficient to confer a high risk for poor pregnancy outcome or if low socioeconomic status and poor pregnancy outcomes are parallel manifestations of dysfunctional maternal characteristics and behaviors. In some instances, this is likely the case. But mothers of low-socioeconomic-status do not invariably have poor pregnancy outcomes; they are merely more likely to than women of higher standing.

Substance Abuse

Maybe drug addicts don't make good parents.[96]
—Karina Bland, *Arizona Republic*, February 1997

Virtually every illicit recreational drug (tobacco and alcohol, too) has been associated with adverse pregnancy outcomes. But due to the many media campaigns against alcohol, tobacco and drugs, it's the rare mother in the

United States who doesn't know that these substances are bad for her and her fetus. Nevertheless, most smoking, drinking or drug-abusing women

156 don't curtail these harmful habits when they're pregnant:

- One in five pregnant women smokes.[97]
- During pregnancy, alcohol may be used by up to 70 percent in some groups and illicit drugs by up to 25 percent.[98, 99]
- One survey revealed that 63 percent of mothers having babies without prenatal care tested positive for alcohol or illicit drugs.[100]
- Drug testing at a large Sacramento, California, hospital revealed a 57-percent rate of alcohol or illegal substance use.[101]
- After a sixteen-year decline in New York City's rate of low-birth-weight babies, a marked increase was noted between 1984 and 1988—coinciding with the introduction of crack cocaine.[102]
- Nationally, the prevalence of alcohol use among pregnant women is on the rise.[103]

Substance abuse varies by age and race/ethnicity. For example, Dr. Constance M. Wiemann at the University of Texas in Galveston found that for all age groups, whites reported higher rates of "lifetime" illicit drug use than Blacks or Mexican-Americans.[104] But Black women twenty-one years of age or older reported the highest rate of current illicit drug use. Interestingly, English-speaking Mexican-American mothers were more likely to report alcohol, tobacco, or illicit drug use than were Spanish-speaking Mexican-American women. In a related study, Dr. Abbey B. Berenson found that Hispanic women with a history of battering were more likely to speak English than Spanish, suggesting that some high-risk behaviors during pregnancy reflect some degree of acculturation to American society.[105]

It's unclear whether substance abuse represents battered victims' attempts to cope with their situation or whether the environment of the substance abuser increases the likelihood that physical abuse will occur. But it's all too clear that presently utilized programs for combating substance abuse during pregnancy have been generally ineffective. For example, a study of over 5,500 mothers in Detroit found that public information campaigns regarding alcohol-related pregnancy risks produced no decrease in maternal drinking.[106] Similarly, Dr. Virginia Lupo found that notifying child protective agencies and offering chemical dependency treatment didn't appreciably reduce substance abuse by mothers during subsequent pregnancies.[107] Even more discouraging is the fact that most prenatal care regimens include no counseling whatsoever regarding how to stop abusing substances, including tobacco.[108]

Stress

Dr. Fredrik F. Broekhuizen at the University of Wisconsin Medical School analyzed the relationship between maternal substance abuse, low birthweight, and adequacy of prenatal care and found that the low birthweight rate was two to three times higher for drug-abusing women who received inadequate prenatal care than for drug abusers who received adequate care.[109] Rather than attributing the differential outcomes of these two groups to the beneficial effects of prenatal care, however, Dr. Broekhuizen concluded that the group with fewer prenatal visits were manifesting greater degrees of "social chaos" in their lives than were substance abusers who were able to maintain their prenatal care appointments. Indeed, Broekhuizen concluded that inadequate prenatal care is a marker of social chaos which may affect pregnancy outcome more than substance abuse itself. However, an equally plausible explanation was offered by the late Dr. Sidney F. Bottoms, who proposed that drug users who receive adequate prenatal care are more likely to be lighter users. In essence, there is less social chaos when drug use is lighter.[110]

When it comes to stress, there is little agreement regarding its definition or quantitation, nor is there consensus regarding its effect on pregnancy outcomes. The causes of stress are also hard to pin down due to their wide-ranging, multifaceted nature: what triggers stress in one person may not in another. Stress can arise acutely from discrete events, build gradually from ongoing problems, or both. Moreover, how one responds to stress can be idiosyncratic and/or difficult to decipher. Intuitively, it would seem that stress should adversely affect pregnancy. Yet untangling the effect of stress from other factors which contribute to prematurity and low birthweight is a daunting task. Highly stressed mothers appear to be at increased risk for a host of problems which themselves may contribute to prematurity or low birthweight. Substance-abusing mothers frequently report high stress levels, but is stress the reason for illicit drug use or is it drugs which are prompting the stress? And isn't pregnancy itself a sufficiently significant "life event" to induce considerable levels of stress? Experts disagree as to whether stress contributes to poor pregnancy outcomes, and if it does, the extent of its effect. A recent review of the topic found fairly mixed results:[111]

158 One study found that higher levels of stress were associated with better pregnancy outcomes.[112] A problem with many studies attempting to relate stress to poor pregnancy outcome is that mothers were frequently queried about prenatal stressors after rather than before delivery. As a result, mothers who delivered premature or low-birthweight infants may have been reflecting the stress of their suboptimal pregnancy outcome instead of prenatal stressors.[113] Alternatively, some may have been seeking to deflect responsibility for poor pregnancy outcome away from themselves (i.e., smoking, drugs, etc.) and onto the more nebulous but socially acceptable concept of "stress." But even if we were to presume that stress is a genuine risk factor for prematurity and low birthweight, it doesn't appear that interventions aimed at reducing stress have been able to consistently reduce prematurity or low birthweight rates.[114] Establishing a pathophysiologic (i.e., biologic) link between stress and poor pregnancy outcome is yet another problem for proponents of the stress-prematurity/low birthweight connection. Some have hypothesized a neuroendocrine link while others have invoked a role for the immune system, but the supporting data is scant.[115–119]

Jail

There may be no greater source of social chaos than a lifestyle that lands a women in jail. As of 1994, there were over 64,000 female prison inmates in the United States; roughly 6 percent of women entering American prisons are pregnant.[120, 121] While the available information regarding incarceration during pregnancy is limited, one would assume that the risk of poor outcomes in this circumstance would be quite high. But recent reports raise the interesting possibility that pregnancy outcomes might actually be improved for women subjected to prolonged incarceration. Reports from Europe have also suggested that pregnant prisoners may actually have better pregnancy outcomes than those allowed to deliver outside of custody.[122–124] Possible contributors to improved outcomes among pregnant inmates may be related to factors that are poorly influenced by contemporary prenatal care: improved nutrition, avoidance of substance abuse, and escape from domestic violence.

To assess the effect of imprisonment upon pregnancy outcome, expectant mothers imprisoned at the Gatesville Unit of the Texas Department of Corrections were studied by Dr. Jason V. Terk of the University of Texas in

Galveston.[125] Dr. Terk found that pregnancy outcomes improved significantly with increasing durations of pregnancy spent in prison. Thus, it appears that enforced cessation of high-risk behavior may have a beneficial effect on maternal and fetal outcome, albeit at a steep price—55,000 dollars per person-year of imprisonment.[126]

    159

In a similar study, Dr. Leandro Cordero at the Ohio State University studied pregnant women serving time at the Ohio Reformatory for Women.[127] This group of women presented many high-risk problems: illegal drug use, tobacco use, as well as obstetrical, medical, and nutritional complications. Nevertheless, Dr. Cordero found that prisoners who had access to well-organized prenatal care and who participated actively in antepartum health education programs during long-term incarceration had better pregnancy outcomes. In yet another report on incarcerated mothers, Dr. Charles Egley of the University of North Carolina analyzed the pregnancy outcomes of women at the North Carolina Correctional Institute for Women, a maximum-security prison.[128] Compared with non-incarcerated mothers, prisoners were less likely to deliver prematurely, to experience premature rupture of the membranes, or to have anemia. Dr. Egley concluded that in addition to prenatal care, the availability of a nutritionally adequate diet, sufficient rest, and sexual abstinence among prisoners (the North Carolina Penal System doesn't allow conjugal visits) might outweigh the detrimental effects of cigarettes and illicit drug use. More recently, Dr. Sandra Martin reviewed the records from the North Carolina Department of Corrections over a five-year period (1987 through 1991).[129] Dr. Martin found that although infant birthweights of women incarcerated during pregnancy were no different from mothers who were never incarcerated, infant birthweights were significantly worse among women jailed at a time other than during pregnancy compared to never-incarcerated women or women jailed during pregnancy. Like other researchers of the topic, Martin concluded that some aspects of the prison environment may be health-promoting for certain pregnant women.

An extension of the above-mentioned studies is the "fetal protection movement," which seeks to put "exposed" fetuses under the jurisdiction of the courts. However, efforts to prosecute women who endanger their fetuses have historically had mixed results. In 1996, the South Carolina Supreme Court let stand the manslaughter conviction of a pregnant woman who shot herself in the abdomen, killing her twenty-week fetus.[130] In 1998, the South Dakota and Wisconsin legislatures passed laws allowing authorities to detain pregnant women who abuse drugs or alcohol, something which Minnesota has quietly permitted since 1988.[131] On the other hand, a California law which would have defined drug use in late pregnancy as criminal child abuse died in committee in 1998. The issue of maternal detention raises a number of difficult issues including:

160

- When it comes to fetal abuse, where does one draw the line (e.g., smoking, failure to obey doctors' orders, etc.)?
- What becomes of the child after delivery?
- Who would be responsible for monitoring pregnant women?

Critics of maternal detention have correctly pointed out that there are not enough slots in treatment programs for pregnant women who come forward voluntarily, let along for those who might be forced there. Moreover, already brimming prisons would be hard-pressed to accept such women, as would most overloaded social service agencies. Critics have also fretted that fears of the "pregnancy police" might prevent some substance-abusing pregnant women from seeking obstetric care, revealing once again the widespread, unfounded faith which we hold in the effectiveness of prenatal care. But there's a lesson to be learned here: much of what causes harm to pregnancies is self-induced. To the extent that mothers can be convinced or coerced to refrain from these activities, there's evidence that their babies will benefit. It's the mother herself who's the final line of defense for her growing fetus. Within this paradigm, it's the mother (and father) who bear much of the responsibility for the well-being of the child. Indeed, it's what mothers choose to avoid that may spell the difference during pregnancy. For a healthy woman, avoidance of drugs, alcohol, tobacco, sexually transmitted disease, and unwanted pregnancy will likely promote better babies better than any number of prenatal visits or well-intended programs.

Race and Culture

The impact of race on pregnancy outcome is both important and complex. Being a member of a minority group may by itself represent a barrier to healthcare access:

- Black patients receive fewer cardiac angiographic screens despite relatively higher rates of coronary disease.[132, 133]

- Despite disproportionate representation on waiting lists for kidney transplants, Blacks are half as likely as whites to receive transplants—and they tend to wait longer for them.[134, 135]
- Between 1986 and 1992, Black Medicare beneficiaries were less likely to undergo coronary bypass procedures than whites and are also less likely to receive seventeen other diagnostic or therapeutic procedures.[136, 137]
- Black Medicare beneficiaries utilize less care and see doctors less frequently than White beneficiaries.[138, 139]

A growing body of data dealing with infant mortality and low birthweight among the country's three largest racial/ethnic groups is beginning to shed light upon the impact of race and ethnicity on pregnancy outcomes. As with other recent research pertaining to race and culture, interesting questions regarding the role of biology, culture, socioeconomic status, and individual behavior as contributors to group differences in perinatal outcome are being raised.

A woman's race/culture appears to affect many pregnancy-related issues. In 1992, for example, 10.9 percent of white women who delivered babies were younger than twenty years, as were 22.7 percent of Black women, 20 percent of Native American women and 5.6 percent of Asian/Pacific Island women.[140] Here in Arizona, the low-birthweight rate of white babies has increased annually since 1980.[141, 142] However, the low birthweight rate among Blacks increased at a two- to fourfold greater rate than for whites—very low-birthweight babies also had their greatest representation among Black newborns.[143] But both Hispanics and Native Americans experienced much lower increases in their low-birthweight rates:[144]

Maternal Characteristics in 1995	Rank Order (High to Low)			
First trimester entry into care	W	B	H	A
Third trimester entry into care	A	H	B	W
No prenatal care	H	A	B	W
1–4 prenatal visits	A	H	B	W
5 or more visits	A	H	W	B
9 or more prenatal visits	W	H	B	A
13 or more prenatal visits	W	B	H	A

A—Native American, B—Black, H—Hispanic, W—White

Reprinted with permission of the Arizona Department of Health Services, from C. K. Mrela. *Arizona Health Status and Vital Statistics, 1995* (Phoenix: Arizona Department of Health Services, 1996).

Despite receiving generally fewer prenatal care visits and fewer early entries into prenatal care clinics, Hispanic and Native American women fared better than Black women in Arizona over the decade of the 1980s and thus far into the '90s with regards to prematurity and low birthweight.[145, 146] Annual surveys of the nation's vital statistics have noted that the proportion of Hispanic-American (largely of Mexican descent) women with low or no prenatal care is similar to that of Black women, but their outcomes with regards to premature and low-birthweight babies is closer to the white population, a phenomenon that's come to be known as the "Mexican Paradox":[147]

	Hispanic	White	Black
Number of births (1991)	623,085	2,589,878	666,758
Late or no prenatal care	11%	3.2%	10.7%
Delivery before 37 weeks	11%	8.7%	19%
Birthweight < 2,500 grams	6.1%	5.7%	13.6%
Birthweight < 1,500 grams	1%	0.9%	3%

Reprinted with permission of *Pediatrics*, from B. Guyer, J. A. Martin, M. F. MacDorman, R. N. Anderson, D. M. Strobino. "Annual Summary of Vital Statistics—1996." *Pediatrics*. 100(1997)905.

More recent data confirms that this relationship is ongoing:[148–150]

	Hispanic	White	Black
Number of births (1996)	701,339	3,093,057	594,781
First trimester entry into care	71.9%	84.0%	71.4%
Birthweight < 2,500 grams	6.3%	6.3%	13%

Reprinted with permission of *Pediatrics*, from B. Guyer, J. A. Martin, M. F. MacDorman, R. N. Anderson, D. M. Strobino. "Annual Summary of Vital Statistics—1996." *Pediatrics*. 100(1997)905, and from B. Guyer, M. F. MacDorman, J. A. Martin, K. D. Peters, D. M. Strobino. "Annual Summary of Vital Statistics—1997." *Pediatrics*. 102(1998) 1333.

In Arizona, the same phenomenon has been noted:[151]

	Hispanic	White	Black
Number of births (1995)	25,141	38,488	2,233
Late or no prenatal care	12.4%	4.6%	8.0%
Delivery (37 weeks)	15.4%	16.2%	21.6%
Birthweight < 2,500 grams	6.6%	6.7%	13.3%
Birthweight < 1,500 grams	1.2%	1.1%	2.6%

Reprinted with permission of the Arizona Department of Health Services, from C. K. Mrela. *Arizona Health Status and Vital Statistics, 1995* (Phoenix: Arizona Department of Health Services, 1996).

Black Women

Underlying causes for differences in pregnancy outcome between the vari-   **163**
ous ethnic groups are complex—a variety of factors are likely at play. Nevertheless, pregnant Black women deserve special mention due to the particularly high-risk status that's been attributed to them. In addition to the Arizona and national statistics, Dr. Saeid B. Amini's analysis of 63,500 deliveries
found that Black women were 30 percent more likely to deliver prematurely
than their white counterparts.[152] A survey of over 5,800 married mothers
conducted by the National Natality Survey from the National Center for
Health Statistics found that for every risk factor reviewed, Black women had
higher rates of preterm birth than did white women. Overall, Black women
had nearly twice the overall rate of prematurity of whites.[153] Through the
decades, the prematurity rate of Black newborns nationwide has been double that of whites and remains so today.[154, 155]

Even when adjusted for maternal age and education level, Black women
still deliver more low-birthweight babies than do white women. Focusing
upon college-educated parents (i.e., those who are supposedly "better off"),
the Centers for Disease Control in Atlanta found that Black infants nevertheless had higher death rates—due largely to higher rates of low birthweight.[156] A study performed in Alameda County, California, suggests that
African-American women may enter the prenatal care system later than white
women, also.[157] African-American women were less likely to start prenatal
care in the first trimester of pregnancy at every level of education and income
and in virtually all categories of financial and insurance status.

Black fetuses may also have distinctly different growth rate patterns which
contribute to some well-known racial differences in pregnancy outcomes. To
illustrate, Dr. Stephen A. Myers at the University of Chicago examined
growth differences between almost 800,000 Black and white newborns in
Illinois from 1980 to 1984.[158] Myers found that fetal growth for both races
is identical until thirty-four weeks gestation, after which time the fetal
growth of Black fetuses decelerates. By the end of pregnancy, the average
birthweight of white babies is over one-half pound heavier than that of Black
newborns. Nevertheless, it's still common to evaluate fetal growth using
"race-neutral," one-size-fits-all criteria—a practice with potentially devastating consequences for Black fetuses. When analyzing fetal growth of
Black and white fetuses using race-neutral criteria, for example, Dr. Myers
found that the stillbirth rate increased significantly among white fetuses
when their body weights fell below the twelfth percentile, whereas Black

fetuses exhibited significantly higher death rates earlier in the process—at the eighteenth percentile, to be exact. In other words, Black fetuses will suffer

164   lethal consequences more often when their growth is evaluated by standards which are more suited to larger white fetuses. Race-neutral criteria may allow a sizable number of babies in potential trouble to slip through the cracks and die. Indeed, Myers found that if the weight of Black fetuses fell to the twelfth percentile (i.e., the danger zone according to race-neutral criteria), a five- to sixfold higher rate of stillbirth would result. He concluded that term Black fetuses were more sensitive to factors that adversely affect growth and that ongoing use of race-neutral data for clinical management of racially mixed populations will not accurately predict their risk of stillbirths. Likewise, a study of over 34,000 births by Dr. Rachel L. Copper at the University of Alabama found that Black fetuses had a significantly increased risk of still-birth when compared to whites (Hispanic women had the lowest stillbirth rate of all).[159]

Fetuses are also at increased risk for prematurity even when only one of their parents is Black. Dr. Melissa M. Adams at the Centers for Disease Control in Atlanta studied more than 1,800 pregnant, active-duty enlisted servicewomen at the four largest United States Army Medical Centers.[160] This population of patients receives fairly uniform prenatal care and is generally more healthy than civilians since each woman must meet health requirements at entry into the military and must also pass annual tests of physical fitness. Because of random drug screening, illicit drug use in this group is relatively low. Therefore, many extraneous issues that often con-found Black and white comparisons may be reduced in this setting. Never-theless, Dr. Adams found that the stillbirth rate among Black women was almost twice that among whites. In addition, the risk for preterm delivery among Blacks was 31 percent higher than that for whites. The increased rate of preterm delivery persisted among mixed-race couples: the risk of prematurity was 31 percent higher than when both parents were white. Very low rates of substance abuse, uniform access to prenatal care, and good maternal health in Dr. Adams study reduced but did not eliminate Black-white differences in prematurity. In another study of this same mili-tary population, Dr. Adams found no difference between Black and white women regarding the prevalence of prenatal hospitalization.[161] Thus, in the absence of social or financial barriers, Black women use the medical system no differently than their white cohorts but experience higher rates of prematurity, nevertheless. Similarly, Dr. James S. Rawlings examined pregnancy outcomes at Madigan Army Medical Center in Tacoma, Washington.[162] Operating under similar safeguards of medical access and quality as those in Dr. Melissa M. Adams' earlier-mentioned study, Dr. Rawlings found that African-American mothers were significantly more likely **165** to deliver prematurely. Rawlings found that whether prematurity was defined as less than thirty-seven, thirty, or twenty-six weeks of gestation, significantly higher rates of delivery were noted among African Americans. Significantly higher rates of low-birthweight and very low-birthweight babies were also noted among African Americans. Fortunately, however, lower rates of Black infant mortality were noted when compared to the civilian Black population.

The Mexican Paradox

Between the 1950s and the 1980s, the United States' infant mortality rate slid from being the sixth best in the world to twenty-second.[163] Between 1950 and 1991, the Black/white infant mortality ratio rose from 1.6 to 2.2, indicating steadily worse outcomes for Black babies.[164] By 1997, the ratio had climbed to 2.3.[165] At the same time, the infant mortality rate for Hispanic-Americans was almost identical to that of whites, despite having economic characteristics (unemployment rate, median income, and education) similar to Blacks. Moreover, this phenomenon occurred despite the fact that Hispanic mothers, mostly of Mexican descent, are no more likely to receive early prenatal care than are Black mothers. Thus, it appears that other factors are contributing to the high rate of suboptimal pregnancy outcomes experienced by Black women.

Dr. Jose E. Becerra at the Centers for Disease Control in Atlanta studied variations in infant mortality among different ethnic groups in the United States for 1983 to 1984.[166] Dr. Becerra also confirmed the twofold increased risk of neonatal death among Blacks, compared to Hispanics or whites. With regards to low-birthweight babies, Dr. Becerra noted that the rate of low birthweight among Black infants was almost 2.5 times higher than the low-birthweight rate of whites. Again, however, no comparable risk was noted for Mexican-American mothers. In 1997, the ratio was still two to one. Becerra also demonstrated that Mexican-American women born in Mexico were less likely to deliver low-birthweight infants than their Mexican-American peers born in the United States.

One study sought to explain the observation that Mexican-American mothers, despite similar socioeconomic disadvantages, have better outcomes than Black mothers. With data from the Hispanic Health and Nutrition

166

Examination Survey, the study's author noted that Mexican-American women with a predominantly Mexican cultural orientation were at lower risk to deliver low-birthweight babies than were Mexican-American mothers who had become "acculturated" to American society.[167] Better outcomes among non-Americanized mothers persisted irrespective of age, education level, income, or smoking status. Thus, it appears that adherence to Mexican culture (or alternatively, resistance to contemporary American culture) conferred perinatal benefit to Mexican-American mothers.

Culture and Tradition

Tradition is not something constant but the product of a process of selection guided not by reason but by success.[168]
—Friedrich A. Hayek, 1973

Dr. Sherman A. James at the University of Michigan posits that Mexican-American mothers with a Mexican orientation derive valuable benefits by maintaining contact with their native culture.[169] He notes that, "Economic disadvantage comes into being as a strong risk factor for low birthweight in U.S. women of color when [they] are no longer adequately 'protected' by the affirming symbols of their native cultures and are simultaneously marginalized (both psychologically and economically) by mainstream U.S. culture."

To study the effect of acculturation on maternal behavior during pregnancy, Dr. Anthony E. Camilli at the University of Arizona studied the differences in tobacco use among Mexican-American and white mothers.[170] Dr. Camilli noted that the odds that Mexican-American mothers would smoke during pregnancy were one-third that of whites. Moreover, the odds of quitting tobacco during gestation were five times higher for Mexican-American mothers who happened to be smokers. In another study of Mexican-Americans, the impact of acculturation regarding smoking behavior was evaluated via an "acculturation score."[171] Mexican-American women who were more "Americanized" were more than twice as likely to smoke as were women with low acculturation scores. Thus, ethnicity as well as acculturation may affect the prevalence of smoking during pregnancy. A similar effect was demonstrated in yet another study on the subject which again found that those who were more Americanized had a higher prevalence of smoking than did less Americanized mothers.[172]

In step with this theme, a report by the Canadian Institute of Advanced Research identified two factors which made important contributions to one's health:[173]

- A greater sense of belonging to a social group.
- Control over one's circumstances and fate.

Perhaps the same factors that have provided protection against suboptimal pregnancy outcome for Mexican-American mothers have, by their undoing among some African-American mothers, placed African-American pregnancies at risk. This phenomenon may in part explain why the rate of low birthweight among foreign-born Black women is one-third lower than that of African-American women.[174, 175] Indeed, one researcher noted that foreign-born Black women giving birth at Boston City Hospital had better pregnancy outcomes than their Black, U.S.-born peers: compared to American-born Black mothers, foreign-born mothers were generally older, more likely to be married, better educated, and less likely to smoke, drink alcohol, or use illicit drugs.[176] Foreign-born Black mothers also tended to have more prenatal care visits than their American-born peers. Even after adjusting for differences in risk factors between foreign-born and American-born Black mothers, the birthweights, body lengths, and head circumferences of babies of Black women were significantly greater among foreign-born Black mothers.

Black infants in other largely non-Black countries don't always lag behind whites when it comes to pregnancy outcomes. In Cuba, for instance, the Black-white disparity in low birthweight and infant mortality is not evident.[177] Likewise, in Sweden, the prematurity rate of Sub-Saharan African immigrants is not significantly different from white Swedish infants, although the rates of low birthweight for white Swedes are still lower.[178] In the mid-1980s, famine and civil war in Ethiopia led to large increases in the number of refugee immigrants to the United States. Haimanot Wasse compared the pregnancy outcomes of women in this group to those of U.S.-born Blacks.[179] During the comparison, Wasse found that family income (as measured by median income census tracts of residence) was similar among Ethiopians and U.S.-born Blacks. In addition, Ethiopian mothers were similar to U.S.-born Blacks in that both groups were less likely than whites to initiate early prenatal care. Nevertheless, Ethiopian-born women were less likely than U.S.-born Black women to deliver low-birthweight infants. In fact, the average birthweight of full-term Ethiopian infants was more similar to that of U.S.-born whites than that of U.S.-born Blacks. Only after adjusting the data for smoking, marital status, and prenatal care (i.e., maternal behavior) did a subgroup of Ethiopians demonstrate a risk for low birthweight similar to U.S.-born Blacks.

Among Wasse's explanations for better pregnancy outcomes among Ethiopian refugees was psychological and emotional (i.e., cultural) support within the local Ethiopian community, a finding repeated in other studies of the topic. Without sound cultural anchoring, many economically disadvantaged mothers may engage in harmful behaviors such as substance abuse despite the knowledge that such activities could adversely effect the well-being of their babies. Irrespective of one's culture, the "norms" fostered generally serve as guidelines that steer women clear of counterproductive or dangerous behavior during gestation. Risk factors, many of which are self-induced, may be minimized by adhering to the strategies (i.e., "traditions") inherent in all cultures that have successfully sustained themselves through time. Most viable cultures have coded within them social or familial mechanisms that ensure propagation of healthy offspring. When asked about the methods they used to stop smoking during pregnancy, for example, 71 percent of Mexican-American women simply replied, "I just quit."[180]

The cultural connectedness of a given prenatal clinic to its clientele may also play a role: low-income (largely Black) mothers receiving prenatal care from nurse practitioners at the Guilford County (North Carolina) Health Department were half as likely to deliver low-birthweight babies as were similar mothers in Guilford County who received prenatal care from private practice physicians who were mostly white.[181] The authors of the study speculated that it was the content of prenatal care visits as well as the type of prenatal care provider that were responsible for the outcomes observed. As suggested by Sherman James at the University of Michigan, the Health Department Clinic likely offered women an "extended, highly knowledgeable female support system . . . much the same way that older, more knowledgeable women have traditionally guided and supported young, inexperienced expectant mothers."[182]

Racism

From the eugenics movement earlier this century to the Tuskegee syphilis study to present-day events, the medical profession's hands have not been entirely clean when it comes to the treatment of minorities. As a result, discussions regarding the effect of racism on pregnancy outcomes are bound to generate more questions than answers, and, frequently, more contention than accord. Among the questions:

How Is Racism Defined and Whose Definition Should We Use? Racism has variously been viewed in terms of economic, social, environmental, or interpersonal discrimination. Thus, obstetricians' historic refusal to see Medicaid patients could be considered implicitly racist since a disproportionate number of Medicaid mothers are non-white. On the other hand, it could be a result of some doctors' unwillingness to accept lower payment rates or to deal with the Medicaid bureaucracy (a situation which seems to be changing as a result of managed care). Still other times, some physicians have not accepted Medicaid patients for fear of running off his/her privately insured clientele. In this scenario, doctors claim that the problem is not their own bias, but their "concern" about the bias of their privately insured patients.

What Are the Effects of Racism upon Pregnancy and How Do We Measure Them? As with stress, there are a number of theoretical ways racism could have its effect, but no clear-cut, widely accepted pathophysiologic mechanism is presently known. The truth is that we don't know what, if any, additional influence racism exerts beyond the factors already at play. In fact, stress itself is frequently cited as the causative agent triggered by racism. From a scientific standpoint, however, this theory has a long way to go before it can be considered a viable explanation. But the stress connection is only one possible pathway to suboptimal pregnancy outcomes; a number of other issues merit consideration, such as how minorities are actually treated by our prenatal care system. For example, a study by Dr. Michael D. Kogan of the National Center for Health Statistics found that pregnant Black women were more likely to report not receiving advice from their prenatal care provider regarding smoking cessation and the dangers of alcohol use.[183] Another study found that pregnant Black women were most likely to be at high medical risk yet were the least likely to actually know what their risk status was, even though Black women in the study were the most highly educated group of subjects.[184] Likewise, a report by Dr. Kate M. Brett of the National Center for Health Statistics found that Black women were significantly less likely to receive or use certain prenatal care technologies such as genetic amniocentesis.[185] But statistical disparities are not necessarily prima facie evidence of discrimination. When it comes to genetic amniocentesis, for example, the procedure is generally performed during the first half of pregnancy, most **170** commonly at approximately sixteen weeks of gestation. Given that a relatively large proportion of African-American mothers do not initiate prenatal care until the third trimester of pregnancy, a disproportionately smaller number of African-American mothers will have the opportunity for genetic testing. But from the perspective of the statistician (or the politician, for that matter), all that will be apparent is a lower rate of amniocenteses among African-American women, and the social implications of that disparity. On the other hand, what a mother is told, how she is told, and when she is told may affect the choices she makes during her pregnancy; moreover, it may influence her perception of the importance of the particular advice she receives, as well as her recall of it. Thus, the nature of the relationship between a pregnant woman and her prenatal care provider may have direct and indirect influences upon the pregnancy.

Why Are the Effects of Racism Not Uniformly Demonstrated across a Given Population? As we have seen, certain minority groups who have experienced discrimination have, in general, fairly good pregnancy outcomes. Asian-Americans, for example, tend to have pregnancy outcomes as good or better than the white majority. Pregnancy outcomes among Hispanics tend to rival those of whites despite the fact that the socioeconomic status of Hispanics is more similar to that of African Americans than to that of whites. Moreover, even among Black women, immigrant Blacks have better pregnancy outcomes than U.S.-born Blacks despite sharing similar socioeconomic status and presumably experiencing similar exposure to racism. Could it be that there are degrees of racism and degrees of responses to racism? Other issues which are frequently overlooked include the fact that African Americans are not a homogenous, monolithic group. In fact, considerable ethnic and socioeconomic diversity exists within the African-American population which may variously protect against or contribute to suboptimal pregnancy outcomes.

Because it is so complex and so fraught with controversy, the width and breadth of the topic preclude a satisfactory exploration when it occupies anything other than the central theme of a study; and in this case, it doesn't. But given the relative ineffectiveness of prenatal care against the myriad issues discussed thus far, it would not seem unreasonable to assume that prenatal care would also have little influence against the effects of racism, whatever they may be.

Pregnancy Wantedness

Unwanted children are at increased risk for many problems, including child 171 abuse and delayed intellectual/social development. Thus, it shouldn't be entirely unexpected that a study of almost 9,000 married pregnant women conducted by Dr. Muhammed N. Bustan at the University of South Carolina demonstrated that unwanted pregnancies were more than twice as likely to result in infants who died during the first twenty-eight days of life.[186] Pregnancy wantedness may also influence maternal behavior during gestation, thereby indirectly affecting the fetus itself. Even in Finland, a nation with generally excellent pregnancy outcomes, unwanted pregnancies are more likely to result in low-birthweight babies.[187]

While policymakers put considerable emphasis on the systematic and economic processes which contribute to the unenviable condition of American prenatal care, the mother's role in the problem is generally ignored. As shown in chapter 3, expansion of Medicaid eligibility for pregnant women isn't necessarily associated with better pregnancy outcomes. Moreover, the failure of such policies was anticipated by M. Schlesinger who noted that, "Requiring the states to expand Medicaid eligibility . . . is likely to yield small improvements in access [and] may well create counterproductive side effects. While financial barriers undoubtedly are important, we believe the relative importance of other attitudes, motivations and constraints on women's behavior during pregnancy has not been adequately assessed."[188]

Attitudinal surveys of mothers who receive inadequate prenatal care report that negative attitudes towards being pregnant discourage prenatal visits. For example, Dr. Marilyn L. Poland at Wayne State University in Detroit analyzed the many barriers to receipt of adequate prenatal care that exist in America.[189] Of six major factors identified, five related to maternal attitudes and behavior:

- Attitudes towards health professionals
- Delays in suspecting pregnancy
- Delay in telling others about their pregnancy
- Misperception of the importance of prenatal care
- Initial attitudes about being pregnant

Likewise, another report observed that women with unwanted pregnancies may initially deny their pregnancies, thereby failing to obtain prenatal care early in pregnancy.[190] In addition, women who obtain late prenatal care or no prenatal care are more likely to have considered abortion.[191] By contrast, women with planned pregnancies are more likely to exhibit behavior conducive to good pregnancy outcomes—outcomes more likely to be associated with early and ample prenatal care. According to Dr. David A. Nagey of the University of Maryland, "It is possible that women destined to have good pregnancy outcome are more likely to seek prenatal care in the first place."[192]

Women who seek early prenatal care may not be actually benefiting from prenatal care itself but from attitudes and behaviors which happen to include prenatal care as part of a personal health regimen. Indeed, the Coronary Drug Research Group found that patients who complied with drug treatment had better outcomes than those who didn't comply, even when the "treatment" was a placebo.[193] Not surprisingly, maternal compliance is much higher in countries with better pregnancy outcomes such as Scandinavia, where prenatal recommendations are followed to such an extent that maternal blood counts may be performed an incredible sixteen times in a given pregnancy despite the absence of anemia—and mothers tend to go along.[194]

To test the proposition that women who want their pregnancies behave differently from those whose pregnancies are undesired, Robert H. Weller at Florida State University studied pregnancy wantedness and prenatal maternal behavior.[195] Compared to smokers with unplanned pregnancies, Weller found that smoking mothers with planned pregnancies were considerably more likely to discontinue smoking. Another report noted that mothers who smoke are less likely to plan their pregnancies than are nonsmokers—nonsmokers are also less likely to consume hard liquor and generally live at a more moderate pace than smokers.[196] Likewise, a study of almost 5,000 Swedish mothers found that women with unwanted pregnancies were more likely to be smokers than those who wanted their pregnancies.[197]

Pregnancy wantedness may also be influenced by socioeconomic status. The Oklahoma Pregnancy Risk Assessment Monitoring System reported higher rates of unintended pregnancy in the United States, especially among low-income women.[198] Specifically, the report demonstrated that among low-income women, 44 percent have unintended pregnancies and 13 percent have pregnancies that are unwanted. The study also found that pregnancy intention varied by a number of maternal factors including: education level, method of payment for obstetric services, smoking status, and the timing of entry into the prenatal care system. In another study of low-income women, only 13 percent stated that they had intended to conceive.[199] Almost nine of every ten women suspected they were pregnant within four months of conception, yet more than one-third still had not initiated prena-

172

tal care by the end of the sixth month of gestation. Acceptance of one's pregnancy, attachment to the fetus, preparatory activities, and a realistic perception of the newborn are part of normal adjustment to gestation.[200] A host of reasons exists for not obtaining prenatal care. In one study of pregnant women who received no obstetric care, nearly half of the reasons given were internal barriers such as depression, unwanted pregnancy, and denial of pregnancy.[201] Among those who deny something as obvious as one's pregnancy, a number of factors have been cited including conflicts around sexuality, rejection of the fetus, and anger towards the baby's father.[202–204] According to Dr. Anna M. Spielvogel of the University of California in San Francisco, denial of an unacceptable reality is a common coping mechanism among some women, including substance abusers, adolescents, and others who might be unprepared or ill-equipped for pregnancy.[205]

In step with the above-mentioned reports, the National Survey of Family Growth demonstrated that women with unwanted pregnancies sought early prenatal care less frequently, had threefold higher rates of Medicaid coverage, and had low-birthweight babies more often than did women with wanted pregnancies.[206] A commentary written in the *Journal of the American Medical Association* noted that women who didn't intend to become pregnant "are at an especially high risk for poor pregnancy outcome . . . will likely fail to seek early pregnancy care and adopt a lifestyle conducive to good pregnancy outcome, and they may not be good caregivers to the children they bear."[207]

In a 1993 letter to the editor of the *Journal of the American Medical Association*, Dr. Bruce Furguson concluded that, "Perhaps it is time to seriously investigate the possibility that prevention of adverse pregnancy outcomes is more likely to be achieved if expanded access to family planning services before pregnancy is combined with expanded Medicaid coverage of prenatal care for pregnancies after they have occurred."[208]

We don't know which components of prenatal care actually increase the prospects for good pregnancy outcomes. But evidence suggests that it may not be prenatal care itself that confers benefit. Rather, the act of seeking prenatal care may in and of itself identify the mother with a personal interest in optimizing the outcome of her child. For highly motivated mothers, if their obstetricians told them to stand on their heads for two hours each day, they probably would; and research could probably demonstrate a correlation between head-standing and better pregnancy outcomes. But in the final analysis, could any reasonable person believe that head-standing was the active ingredient that produced better babies?

It's the woman who actively seeks prenatal care who's more likely to engage in other health-promoting behaviors. Frequently, women who receive no prenatal care avoid it because of drug addiction, alcoholism, or transient lifestyle. Such behaviors may be manifestations of unhealthy attitudes that permeate all aspects of some women's lives. Therefore, it's not surprising that the woman who seeks care is less prone to substance abuse during pregnancy. She's also more likely to be well-nourished, well-rested and to generally refrain from behaviors that may be detrimental to her baby's well-being. Thus, it may not be the care but the care-seeker that makes the difference. Conversely, the woman who doesn't seek prenatal care may be telling us about her attitude regarding her pregnancy. A British study investigated the attitudes of women who had previously delivered low-birthweight babies, finding that nearly four in ten did not see low birthweight as a problem.[209] Yet six in ten of these women said their babies had been in an intensive care unit and seven of ten said their children had difficulties after delivery. Moreover, 15 percent did not believe that their babies were developing normally and over 40 percent said they had ongoing concerns about their children's development. According to Dr. Marilyn L. Laken at Wayne State University in Detroit, "It may be that prenatal care is valued by women because they believe it contributes to their health and the health of the fetus. This may be sufficient incentive to keep most prenatal appointments."[210]

Interpregnancy Interval

There appears to be a relationship between the amount of time which elapses between a woman's pregnancies and her risk for delivering a premature baby. Specifically, women conceiving within three months of their last delivery seem to be at greatest risk.[211, 212] Among those waiting at least nine months, the danger diminishes markedly.[213] The medical basis for this phenomenon is unclear. Generally, a woman's physiologic function reverts to its baseline, non-pregnant state (with the exceptions of body weight, muscle tone, and aerobic fitness) within six weeks of delivery. Whether an extremely short interpregnancy interval is a proxy for other contributors to prematurity—pregnancy wantedness, for example— is unknown. Clearly, there are some families who want their children closely spaced, but given that child spacing implies a certain degree of planning, it is not unreasonable to assume that foreshortened interpregnancy intervals are often the products of unplanned/unwanted pregnancies and the associated issues and problems which accompany them.

Abortion

The *U.S. Government World Fact Book* cites Japan's infant mortality rate as among the lowest in the world.[214] A study from the University of Rochester searched for factors which may explain the low infant mortality rate in Japan. Among eight factors identified was access to abortion services.[215] With the premise that unwanted pregnancies are the pregnancies most likely to be aborted, Dr. Mark I. Evans at Wayne State University in Detroit studied the impact of a Medicaid abortion ban in Michigan.[216] In December 1988, a "no Medicaid funding of abortion" law went into effect in his state. Thereafter, the number of abortions in Michigan dropped by roughly 10,000 annually. Over the same period, the percentage of NICU admissions for Medicaid babies at Dr. Evans' hospital rose by more than 6 percent. Evans' study suggests that pregnancy unwantedness may give rise to NICU admissions which may have been avoided had access to abortion services been an option. In support of this theory is the fact that the steepest decline in America's low-birthweight and neonatal mortality rates were roughly coincident with the legalization of abortion nationwide in the early 1970s.[217] A 1984 study found that states which did not fund abortions for low-income women had to spend greater amounts to cover maternity care, healthcare for the infant, AFDC, and nutritional support for women on Medicaid.[218] The study concluded that for every dollar spent on abortions for poor women, four dollars were purportedly saved in medical and welfare costs over the ensuing two years. Within the context that all arguments based on the "for-every-dollar-spent" tactic should be viewed with caution, one must consider if pregnancy outcomes and the greater social good would not be helped by reducing the number of unwanted pregnancies in our nation. The larger question, however, is whether wholesale abortion is the method for achieving it.

According to Dr. Kenneth J. Meier at the University of Wisconsin, a one-dollar-per-capita increase in family planning expenditures is associated with one less abortion per 1,000 women.[219] Dr. Meier also found that in states that funded abortions, there were nearly 152,000 fewer births to teenagers, 21,300 fewer premature births, and almost 233,000 fewer births with late or no prenatal care. Two other studies also found that availability of abortion services was associated with lower rates of low-birthweight babies.[220, 221]

But the point here is not to showcase the utility of abortion, it is to demonstrate the effect of pregnancy wantedness upon pregnancy outcomes. Even

176 when adoption is chosen over abortion, pregnancy outcomes appear to be at increased risk for being suboptimal.[222] Indeed, a study of mothers who selected adoption demonstrated significantly higher rates of prematurity and low birthweight despite the fact that they were given housing and biweekly prenatal monitoring once adoption arrangements had been made.

Abortion as a social tool is one more example of the assumption that medicine can provide a simple remedy for our social ills. America's abortion rate already outstrips Australia's and Western Europe's (i.e., places with generally better pregnancy outcomes than ours). Only China, Cuba and the former Eastern Bloc countries perform more. While abortion is one possible solution to our maternity woes, it is a desperate one; one which merely sweeps our underlying social and cultural problems under the rug. Indeed, it has not escaped notice that minority women are vastly over-represented among those undergoing pregnancy termination: the abortion rate for Black women, for example, is nearly triple that of whites. An extreme view of this phenomenon is that abortion represents a type of immigration control for individuals, disproportionately minority, who enter our nation from the womb. Yet the fact remains that abortion is something which is chosen. It is unclear (but tragically American), however, why women would choose an option which is multifold more risky and costly than a conscientiously followed regimen of contraception.

Counterpoint

In our efforts to solve the prematurity problem, a remarkable proliferation of research has identified an impressive array of risk factors. Based on these studies, one might conclude that a fairly accurate picture could be painted of the mother most at risk for premature delivery (i.e., a poor, unmarried African-American teenager who smokes, uses drugs, has sexually transmitted diseases, and is physically abused by her partner, for example), a notion which holds a certain medical and political allure for some. But to do so would be to ignore the fact that obstetric risk profiles have utterly failed to reliably identify those destined for premature delivery. Why? In part, our failure is a reflection of our incomplete understanding of the problem. In part, we fail because we tend to look at risk factors in a vacuum with little regard to the prevalence of the risk factor (teen pregnancy, for example) in the population or how the risk factor is modified by other patient characteristics and environmental conditions. As Dr. Paul H. Wise of Harvard University points out, the elimination of teenage pregnancies in America would reduce infant mortality by only about 10 percent.[223] Indeed, while the teen pregnancy rate has fallen in each of the last six years, our nation's low-birthweight rate has climbed higher than it has been in decades.[224] Even if a pregnant woman exhibited all known high-risk features for prematurity, it would not guarantee a premature delivery. In fact, one study which focused on birthweight found that less than 10 percent of the variation in birthweight was explained by more than forty risk factors which were examined.[225] While one must not conclude that risk factors carry no weight, the fact remains that at least half of America's low-birthweight babies come from mainstream adult women who harbor no risk factors and who have had at least some prenatal care.

Adding to the problem, doctors appear to interact differently with patients of different socioeconomic levels, giving varying amounts of information in relation to patient age, sex, income, and education level.[226] Patients who are upper-middle class, middle-aged, more seriously ill, or more highly educated tend to receive more information from their doctors than do patients who lack these characteristics.[227] For instance, one study found that doctors are more likely to justify their treatment choices to college-educated patients than they are to less educated patients.[228, 229]

Rebuttal

Although a pregnant woman is not generally considered to be a mother until after she has delivered her child, I have nevertheless referred to expecting women in this book as mothers for the following reasons.

For the Woman Who Chooses to Continue with Her Pregnancy, Her Maternal Role Begins at Conception, Not at Delivery. There are few times in a woman's life when she will be as motivated to modify her behavior as she will be during pregnancy. Thus, the woman who fails to abstain from unhealthy or counterproductive activity during or in preparation for pregnancy may be even less likely to do so afterwards. Not only is healthful behavior during pregnancy generally inexpensive, some aspects of it are free or money-saving; avoiding alcohol, tobacco, or drugs, for example, would actually put money back into a mother's pocket. For those who subscribe to the notion that simply stopping or avoiding such harmful activities is unrealistic, they must accept the equally unrealistic belief that the benefits of prenatal care override the harmful effects of unhealthy habits during pregnancy. Alternatively, one could advocate preventing or delaying childbearing, especially among unmarried or teen-aged women. However, a certain amount of caution would be advised regarding this strategy, as well. A report by the Robin Hood Foundation, for example, compared pregnant teenagers who delivered babies and those who miscarried, finding very little difference in the education level ultimately achieved or in earnings.[230] The results of the report raise the question of whether avoiding pregnancies in at-risk populations improves things or merely keeps already unstable situations from getting worse.

A Woman's Prenatal Attitudes and Behaviors Correlate with Her Attitudes and Behaviors in General. The unmarried, unmotivated, or otherwise ill-prepared pregnant woman brings more than mere gestation to her prenatal care provider. She brings a host of psychosocial and intangible factors which predate her pregnancy. Some would suggest that single parenthood increases the likelihood for low socioeconomic status (or vice versa). But an equally plausible explanation is that factors like single parenthood and low socioeconomic status are not related in a linear fashion (i.e., one does not necessarily lead to the other). Instead, these two factors may simply represent different facets of a given mother's life/lifestyle which are not helped by a short course of prenatal care. According to Dr. Susan E. Mayer, author of *What Money Can't Buy*, the long-term poor tend to be different from the non-poor: "When families fall on hard times and stay there for years, this means they cannot or will not find a way to support themselves. The children in such families often need outside help that goes beyond economic support."[231] By extension, these families/mothers are more likely to be at risk for poor pregnancy outcomes, not just because they are poor but because of the associated problems which lead to and sustain poverty. Dr. Mayer's thesis is that the traits that make a person a good employee (e.g., reliability, diligence, good health, etc.) probably also make them better parents, and again by my extension, better parents during pregnancy.

Dr. Mayer's review of data from the PSID (Panel Study of Income Dynamics) would suggest that parental factors become more important than income with regards to the outcome of their children, once their basic needs have been met. Indeed, most poor American families meet their basic necessities through a combination of programs such as Food Stamps, housing subsidies, Medicaid, WIC, et cetera. In excess of $11,000 in government benefits (benefits which go uncounted in statistics on income) are distributed to poor households in America.[232] The federally funded Women, Infants and Children (WIC) Food Supplement Program also provides nutritional support to poor women, spending over $2 billion for 4.5 million persons in 1990, for an average expenditure of almost $470 per recipient (producing no reduction in the rate of low-birthweight babies in a study by Dr. Haywood Brown at Indiana University Medical Center).[233, 234] As of 1996, welfare recipients in five states and the District of Columbia were paid the equivalent of a twelve-dollar-per-hour job, while seventeen states provided benefits worth ten dollars per hour.[235] Forty-seven states provided welfare benefits which exceeded the starting salary of a janitor, twenty-seven paid more than the mean starting salary for a secretary, and nine exceeded the first-year salary for teachers.[236] Moreover, the poor spent an average of $1.94 for every dollar of income.[237] Dr. Mayer asserts that in this situation, the things which most favorably affect children cost very little and depend less on income than they do on parental attitudes and behaviors.

By extension to pregnancy, once a mother's basic necessities have been provided, it is up to her to steer clear of trouble, at least of the self-induced variety. Dr. Barbara M. Aved found that 95 percent of patients she surveyed expressed the belief that prenatal care was very or considerably important and should be started early.[238] However, nearly three in ten did not even try to obtain prenatal care. Some studies have also suggested that premature babies at risk for abuse at home can be identified before the children even leave the hospital, based on differences in the nursery visiting behaviors of the parents.[239] In one study, these differences were unrelated to distance from the nursery or the incidence of maternal medical complications (i.e., things which would prevent mothers from visiting). According to one researcher, infrequent nursery visits may be one manifestation of preexisting factors which place these children at risk.[240] Thus, it would not seem unreasonable that in some cases, certain maternal attitudes, situations, or behaviors were also at play during the prenatal period which may have influenced the ultimate outcome.

Should we blame the victim when bad outcomes occur? Sometimes the plight of a child is the fault of its mother. The mother isn't the victim in this scenario, her baby is. Even if we could eliminate all dysfunctional prenatal activities, prematurity would still persist as a problem, albeit at a lower rate. But the point remains: much of what promotes better pregnancy outcomes has less to do with prenatal care than it does with caring during the prenatal period. To an extent, the omission of counterproductive maternal behavior may outweigh (or at least compliment) the commission of certain supposedly beneficial activities at the hands of obstetricians. To be clear, poor pregnancy outcomes are not usually the fault of mothers, nor are all (or even most) women with suboptimal pregnancy outcomes bad mothers. Indeed, the issue is less about maternal culpability than it is about the inability of prenatal care to counteract the aggregation of factors—recognized and unrecognized—which contribute to prematurity. We cannot ignore and must address the issues raised in this chapter; but ultimately, it is not about profiling those most at risk for prematurity—we know that maternal risk analysis has been a failure. Even if we could pinpoint those destined for premature delivery, the fact would remain that prenatal care does little to prevent this all-too-common pregnancy complication, nor does it do anything to remedy the underlying antecedent problems which sometimes accompany and contribute to a mother's pregnancy outcome.

What We Can Do about It: Step Five

1. Greater Parental Accountability for Pregnancy and Pregnancy Outcomes

No system, however well designed, will be effective if individuals do not participate in a reasonable, responsible fashion. Ample, excellent prenatal care cannot compensate for unhealthy maternal behavior. The woman who does not wish to become pregnant should take steps to avoid pregnancy—no one can do it for her. Whether she intends to give her child up for adoption or not, the woman who chooses to carry a pregnancy should do her utmost to optimize her child's outcome—no one can do that for her, either. Even if prenatal care is not sought, there are many healthy behaviors which are inexpensive and sustainable. Moreover, they are behaviors encouraged by most cultures and advised by virtually every media form in this country. The effect of pregnancy wantedness has already been discussed, but its importance can't be overstated. Babies don't just happen—parents must take greater responsibility for the timing of each pregnancy as well as the environment into which each newborn is brought. This is hardly a new idea—the notion of family planning is decades old. But even from a strictly socioeconomic basis, the benefits of delayed childbearing, of fewer children, and of pregnancies that are actually intended (i.e., "planned") become clear: having fewer children reduces the likelihood of poverty in a family.[241]

At the center of American prenatal care is the American mother. In the midst of many economic and political forces that influence prenatal care in this country, the pregnant woman plays a role that is too often minimized. The well-being of a mother and her fetus can be affected by her own behavior. Indeed, a considerable share of illness among women (and men, for that **181** matter) is directly or indirectly self-induced. Malignancies of the skin and lungs as well as many cardiovascular abnormalities are examples of life-threatening disease, the incidence of which would be dramatically reduced by behavioral changes. The problem is that self-destructive behavior such as smoking is far removed in time for the consequence of lung cancer or emphysema. Moreover, the offending behavior is frequently enjoyable to the person. Prenatal care, however earnest or plentiful, cannot compensate for dangerous or counterproductive practices. On the other hand, the healthy mother who takes care of herself can weather the changing political tides of American healthcare and even a considerable amount of systematic neglect. We give prenatal care undue credit. The expectant mother does not receive an extra portion of "health" by entering the contemporary obstetrical system any more than visits to the dentist on a weekly basis confers improved dental health beyond what a good diet and regular brushing provides. Human reproduction is a system that has been fine-tuned through evolution. To the extent that we do not compromise a healthy pregnancy with abuse or neglect, the fetus will sustain itself. Whether she seeks the care of a midwife or obstetrician, the healthy, motivated woman will optimize her chances for achieving a good pregnancy outcome if she avoids alcohol, tobacco, drugs, and sexually transmitted diseases, gets plenty of rest, eats well, and exercises moderately—essentially the same formula for health that applies to all people, pregnant or not.

The recognition of a child's right to recover legal damages for prenatal injury is generally considered to pertain to physician liability. Less frequently acknowledged—but no less valid—is the issue of parental liability for negligently induced prenatal injury. The California Court of Appeals alluded to the possibility of parental liability for "wrongful life" in 1980: "no sound public policy . . . should protect those parents from being answerable for the pain, suffering and misery which they have wrought upon their offspring."[242]

American courts are unanimous in their recognition of a child's right to pursue civil action against a third party for negligently/intentionally inflicted prenatal injury. Historically, parents have not been included in this group. However, this situation may be changing. In 1987, an Illinois Appellate Court found that a five-year-old girl could pursue tort action against her mother for prenatal injuries sustained in an automobile accident that occurred during gestation, thereby recognizing that parents are not immune from suits by their children.[243] In 1980, a Michigan court of appeals determined that a mother who had been unreasonable in her behavior during pregnancy could be held liable by the child, just as any third party could be if they engaged in negligent behavior.[244] As such, the Michigan case was the first to recognize that civil remedies could be applied to parents who negligently injure their fetuses. But as noted by Dr. Lynn D. Fleisher at the 1987 conference of the Health Law Institute of DePaul University College of Law:

> In the very unique circumstances of pregnancy, the conflicts that arise from the recognition of a prematernal duty are compelling. They involve, on the one side, the right of the child to be born free of any negligently induced injury, and on the other side, the constitutionally guaranteed right of the pregnant women to personal privacy and bodily integrity under Roe v. Wade. . . . The question of whether a pregnant woman has a legally enforceable duty to act non-negligently to protect the health of a fetus she apparently intends to carry to term is not an easy one to answer.[245]

Nevertheless, the issue of civil (and in some instances, criminal) liability on the part of negligent parents is an issue that will likely receive more attention in the coming years.

2. Paternal Responsibility

No aspect of prenatal care has been more ignored than the father's responsibility for ensuring optimal pregnancy outcome. The emotional, logistical, and economic support that a father may provide is invaluable. The concept that prenatal care is a commodity bestowed by an obstetrician undermines the benefit that a healthy, stable lifestyle provides. The role the father can play to encourage appropriate maternal behavioral changes and to provide assistance is extremely important. Yet there are other benefits to be had from a stable, supportive, monogamous relationship during pregnancy. The reduced incidence of sexually transmitted disease and substance abuse that is generally associated with such relationships is also associated with lower incidence of premature and low-birthweight babies.

The principles of paternal responsibility that pertain to divorced fathers should also apply to uninvolved fathers of fetuses. While proof of paternity may need to wait until after childbirth, biologic fathers should be economically accountable for part or all of their child's prenatal and neonatal care expenses. Indeed, the same enforcement techniques currently applied to delinquent fathers should apply to the prenatal period as well. To this end, the father's social security number should be printed on a newborn's birth certificate. The utility of male sterilization should also be fostered. Compared to female sterilization techniques, the vasectomy is quicker, cheaper, and safer.[246] Despite vasectomy's clear-cut advantages, however, contraception and sterilization have unfortunately been the historic responsibility of women.

183

3. Aggressive Family Planning

More than half of all pregnancies in this nation are unintended.[247] As such, contraception has the potential to play a vital role in the prevention of unintended babies, especially in light of the fact that the average cost of each pregnancy exceeds $3,000 in a managed care setting.[248] *The Medical Herald*, an urban medical newspaper, recently conducted a survey to assess women's attitudes towards contraception.[249] The results of the survey found a number of reasons for the growing trend—especially among minority women—away from contraception:

- *Religion.* Despite recent reform efforts, church opposition to contraception and abortion services appears to have intensified.
- *Economics.* Paradoxically, many women cite financial barriers to contraception despite the fact that the cost of raising a child is many times more expensive than birth control.
- *Suspicion and Misunderstanding.* According to the *Medical Herald*, superstition, rumor, and fear play a role in the growing reluctance to use contraceptives. For example, a small segment of Hispanic women have been advised that contraceptives are a "white man's plot" to limit the number of births in this group. Moreover, recent lawsuits against contraceptive manufacturers have fostered the notion that birth control is unsafe.
- *Lack of Knowledge.* A distressing number of women still know very little about contraceptive/family planning options and how to pursue them.

Given the influence of pregnancy wantedness upon pregnancy outcome, it would seem that an important aspect of prenatal care is to ensure that we maximize the proportion of pregnancies that are wanted. According to the Alan Guttmacher Institute, "Initiation of sexual intercourse during the teenage years has become the norm in the United States. . . . More than eight in ten adolescents have had intercourse by the time they are 20. . . . As sex has become more common at younger ages, historic differences in sexual activity among different races, income levels and religions have narrowed considerably."[250] Mary Mahowald of University of Chicago notes that the growing problem of unwanted pregnancies "is a matter of class rather than color."[251] For example, 60 percent of poor women aged fifteen to nineteen are sexually active while 53 percent of low-income and 50 percent of high-income teenagers are sexually experienced. At the same time, the rate of unplanned pregnancies among poor women under age twenty are appreciably higher in the United States than in other developed nations despite similar patterns of sexual activity.[252, 253]

Exemplifying our undue faith in prenatal care and our disregard for responsible behavior, Josie Morales, senior director of women's health programs of the New York City Health and Hospitals Corporation, points out how the media refuses to carry public service announcements that address family planning and contraception:

> The public TV network ran an entire series on women's health issues, but they specifically omitted anything related to family planning—let alone abortion—and they did this despite the objections and protests of many women's health groups. They are running stuff on pregnancy, but they are not running anything on family planning, contraception, abortion and all of those things that are a part of the preventive healthcare services to women.[254]

According to Dr. Felicia H. Stewart, Deputy Assistant Secretary for Population Affairs at the United States Department of Health and Human Services, only 10 percent of reproductive-age women consistently refuse to use contraception.[255] However, this group accounts for almost 50 percent of all unintended pregnancies, representing roughly 1.7 million pregnancies annually. Dr. Stewart notes, "The average cost of an unplanned pregnancy is about 3,000 dollars. . . . When you stop and think about it . . . any method of contraception is a bargain."[256] Within this context, work by Dr. James Trussell at Princeton University demonstrates that even the most expensive forms of contraception are bargains compared to the cumulative costs of using no birth control.[257] The cumulative five-year costs for various forms of

184

contraception were as follows: tubal ligation—$2,584, vasectomy—$763, and birth-control pill—$1,784. Of note, the costs of tubal ligation and vasectomy were basically the costs of performing the procedures. Thereafter, **185** expenses were essentially zero. By comparison, the cumulative five-year cost of using no contraception was $14,663. As Dr. Trussell notes:

> The problem that exists now in this country is that there is a disconnect between who pays for contraception and who pays for unintended pregnancies. The cost of contraceptives is usually paid by individuals, not health insurance companies. But insurance companies, by and large, usually pay for spontaneous [miscarriages], ectopic pregnancies and deliveries. . . . It seems to us that a lot of people who run managed care plans are going to sit up and take notice when they compare the modest cost of contraception with the extremely high cost of unintended pregnancy.[258]

Another aspect of contraception that has impeded access to reliable birth control is the requirement that birth-control pills be dispensed by prescription only. There are five criteria for establishing the need for some drugs to be regulated:[259]

- There is difficulty diagnosing the condition for which the drug is given.
- The drug's dosage requires frequent adjusting.
- There is a narrow margin between a drug's therapeutic and toxic doses.
- Overdose of the drug is harmful.
- The drug is addictive.

Some have recommended that women's preventive health screenings such as Pap smears remain linked to physicians prescribing of birth-control pills to maintain compliance. However, Dr. David A. Grimes duly notes:

> Preventive health services are important in their own right and should not be an appendage of contraception. Stated alternatively, women should not have contraception held hostage because of unrelated screening tests, especially when the results will not influence the decision about oral contraception. As one observer wryly noted, "Should a man's purchase of condoms from a pharmacy be contingent upon a digital rectal examination for prostate cancer?"[260]

186

Those in favor of regulating birth-control pills express concerns that without physician counseling, compliance would be adversely affected.[261] As with prenatal care, however, there is little evidence that busy physicians currently spend much time counseling their patients. As nine of the ten most popular over-the-counter medications in the United States were originally available by prescription only, there seem to be steadily fewer reasons not to facilitate access to this effective contraceptive method.[262] Indeed, epidemiologists and family planning experts agree that on safety grounds, one could justify over-the-counter status for low-dose oral contraceptives.[263] At present, however, support for non-prescription birth-control pills is not widespread, even among American women. A recent Gallup Poll found that 86 percent of women surveyed in the United States believe that birth-control pills are too dangerous for over-the-counter use, underscoring the worrisome findings of the Medical Herald survey mentioned earlier.[264, 265]

Why do so many women believe oral contraception is dangerous? One significant contributor to this misperception is the popular press. To illustrate, Morton A. Lebow of the American College of Obstetricians and Gynecologists investigated how four of our nation's largest newspapers (*The New York Times*, *The Washington Post*, *The Chicago Tribune*, and *The Los Angeles Times*) reported on nine major studies of the health effects of oral contraceptives in the eleven-year span between 1986 and 1997.[266] Although all nine studies showed no increased risk of breast cancer and/or actual protective effects against ovarian and uterine cancer, only one of the studies was reported by all four major newspapers. Among the other eight studies, when any mention was made at all, it was usually made by only one of the four publications and typically on the back pages. Other times, the generally benign or beneficial effects of the pill were reported with a negative slant. For example, in 1989, the Food and Drug Administration (FDA) convened a panel to determine if the labeling of oral contraceptives needed to be changed in view of three studies that found connections with breast cancer in several discrete groups of women. Ultimately, the FDA panel decided against labeling changes. Even so, *The Washington Post* headlined the story, entitled, "FDA Panel to Consider Pill Warnings," on its front page. The story's subhead was "New Studies Suggest Breast Cancer Link." However, the follow-up story which reported the FDA panel's decision was printed on page nine. Meanwhile, *The New York Times* used the FDA hearings as the "hook" for launching four days of front-page articles regarding the fear of the connection between breast cancer and oral contraceptives, despite the fact that *The Times* had given superficial coverage to only two of the nine favorable studies of the pill published between 1986 and 1997. Mr. Lebow concluded in his study that "The health consequences of unbalanced reporting of the effects of oral contraceptives can be severe, as shown by the high rate of unintended pregnancy in the United States." Mr. Lebow's comment is supported by a 1980 report in the journal, *Family Planning Perspectives*, which noted that after any unfavorable story about any contraceptive method, discontinuation rates of those methods rose.[267] In the words of Cristine Russell (as quoted by Mr. Lebow), special health reporter for *The Washington Post*, "Exposure to media coverage of women's health risks can itself be hazardous to one's health if those who create the news and those who cover it are not prepared to do a balanced, accurate and informative job of presenting a given problem."

During pregnancy, it is the duty of the prenatal care provider to present each mother with all clinical management options. This rule also applies to available family planning options. Many family planning experts suggest that a component of any program to end the welfare cycle should include the provision of family planning education and services to women who cannot afford to become pregnant. This would seem especially pertinent in an era of shrinking payouts to "welfare mothers." Surveying conservative Republicans and liberal Democrats alike, the *Medical Herald* found that new legislation to encourage the use of contraceptives to reduce the costs of supporting unwed mothers and their children—now in excess of thirty billion annually—is not even being contemplated.[268] According to one U.S. Congressman's office, "There is no pending legislation (on contraception or family planning) that we are sponsoring or co-sponsoring." Instead, his concerns centered around "making sure that pregnant teenagers have access to prenatal care and other services they need."[269]

As we have seen, one factor which influences a mother's response to pregnancy is whether the baby was planned or desired. Within this context, all sexually active women who do not desire pregnancy should use contraception. Every man or woman with two children should be made aware of the availability of permanent sterilization.

6. A Thin Line

The objective of prenatal care is essentially the same throughout the industrialized world. Yet it is in the United States, where care is provided with such high-tech flourish, that pregnancy outcomes are among the worst. We spend more for it, provide more of it, and have intensified it more than any nation on earth. In return, our prematurity, low-birthweight, and very low-birthweight rates have accelerated. Some characterize our problem as a social disease, the biologic expression of a culture run amok. At the very least, it represents the final common pathway for a multitude of contributing factors, most of which cannot be overcome or compensated by prenatal care. Indeed, if the essence of prenatal care could be distilled into a drug, the Food and Drug Administration would likely not approve it due to the lack of effectiveness. Thus, faced with the choice of eliminating counterproductive parental behavior or American prenatal care in its present form, one could argue that we would be marginally better served by discarding the latter.

If prenatal care does little to avert our most dreaded pregnancy complications, what is to become of it? How we answer this question will impact the way prenatal care is provided in the future, how it is funded, and perhaps most importantly, how it is perceived. Depending on one's point of view, prenatal care is

A Cost-Saving Endeavor. The best criterion by which to judge prenatal care is whether it produces better outcomes, and most of the data suggests that it doesn't. If popular support for prenatal care is based upon the premise that prenatal care is cost-effective, support may wane if this premise proves to be incorrect, as I believe it has. A system of care predicated upon cost-effectiveness and not clinical effectiveness will produce neither.

Our Moral Obligation. We live in interesting times. That prematurity persists as the central issue in perinatal and neonatal medicine is the fault of everyone and no one. Advocates of our prenatal care system build their careers endorsing well-intended measures that do not necessarily benefit pregnant women. Meanwhile, there is little pay-off for policymakers to encourage responsible behavior on the part of their constituents. Instead, wholehearted support is given to ever more grandiose prenatal programs, addressing the issues of illegitimacy and pregnancy wantedness only after the fact. But policymakers don't have to make things better; they merely have to make policy. In the final analysis, therefore, it is more important to be perceived as doing something than it is to ensure that real benefit is accruing. Is it moral to offer placebos to our patients? Conversely, would it be immoral to deny them?

A Cure in Search of a Disease. Medicalized prenatal care has been no more able to surmount the societal ills which contribute to America's poor pregnancy outcomes than emergency rooms have been able to solve our nation's violent crime problem. The perception of pregnancy as a disease necessarily produces a system of prenatal care which is decidedly medicalized, intrusive, and largely unsuited for the vast majority of pregnant women. Whatever form prenatal care takes in the future, the vast majority of pregnant women will still have gratifying outcomes. At the same time, a small number will fare poorly, irrespective of the care received. The goal, therefore, will be to minimize the number of women who fall victim to the system itself. A highly technical prenatal system such as ours is bound to salvage some babies. But in its wake will be a considerable number who are harmed or not helped by unnecessary interventions (especially if the effectiveness of the interventions is overestimated so as to increase the likelihood they will be used). Conversely, a passive, overly staid philosophy will produce less unnecessary meddling but will also result in a considerable number who might have been helped by intervention, had it been offered. Therefore, the task for care providers will be to establish a level of care that reduces the frequency of injury which can arise from acts of omission or commission. When it comes to medical vigilance during pregnancy, where we set the bar is merely a matter of opinion. But experience would suggest that our present system of prenatal care has become so medicalized, it is like a cure in search of a disease—a disease which most women don't have.

A Boat Best Not Rocked. Maternity care is a multibillion dollar industry. Attempts to modify it will not be easy. Obstetricians will not relinquish their role without a fight, nor can our prenatal system do without them until workforce transitions have occurred. Despite the fact that obstetricians and nurse-midwives produce pregnancy outcomes that are equivalent, obstetricians will not likely accept the same level of reimbursement as midwives. Many American women who have become accustomed to medicalized care will not likely accept nurse-midwives as mainstream prenatal care providers initially; nor will they welcome the news that many aspects of prenatal care are overrated, understudied, or worthless.

An Opportunity. The certitude with which the benefit of prenatal care has been espoused has neither been supported by medical science nor by our nation's collective experience over the past forty years. Thus, one must conclude that although prenatal care is desirable, the contemporary iteration is somewhat less than crucial when it comes to preventing prematurity and a host of other pregnancy complications, as well. But there is a thin line between downgrading our opinion of prenatal care and calling for its elimination. The purpose of *Expecting Trouble* has been to sound the alarm, not to wave the white flag. Nevertheless, if prenatal care does not produce the results we've been led to believe it does, should it be publicly funded as generously as it has been, or should private patients be expected to pay what they have been paying? Should federal law continue to mandate that insurance companies cover it, and should we continue expanding Medicaid eligibility for it? Whatever the future brings, we should not impede access to prenatal care. But at the same time, the nature of prenatal care should change. Among the changes, there should be a lowering of expectations among mothers and caregivers alike, including the acknowledgment that:

- Our diagnostic and therapeutic armory is smaller and less effective than most realize.
- In the present cultural, economic, and medicolegal climate, what a pregnant woman gets from the American healthcare system is frequently not what she needs.
- To the degree that prenatal care's contribution to pregnancy outcome shrinks, the mother's relative contribution grows.

When uncomplicated pregnancies are medicalized, prenatal care is perceived to be a curative endeavor. Having been shown that this scenario is incorrect, however, our perception of prenatal care must also change. A more realistic, pragmatic view of prenatal care is that it simply represents an opportunity which is available to motivated pregnant women which, in a less medicalized system:

191

- Would allow most women to avoid needless and costly meddling.
- Would replace the bells and whistles of the world's most expensive prenatal care with the time, interaction, and education which most American mothers' healthcare dollars have been unable to buy in the present system.
- Would still not counteract the ill effects of most self-induced harm.
- Would still not reduce the incidence of most pregnancy complications.
- Would allow detection of certain pathologic processes so as to facilitate referral to an appropriate level of care where their outcomes may possibly be optimized.
- Will probably be the system through which genuine advances in prenatal care will reach pregnant women in the future.

A Word about Maternal-Fetal Specialists

Over the course of this book, obstetricians have been criticized at practically every turn. To be clear, our present state of affairs is not the fault of America's obstetricians; the problem is that they cannot make things better. If prenatal care can be provided which is of equal quality, produces equal or greater patient satisfaction, and which is less invasive and more economical than that provided by obstetricians, why should pregnant women not avail themselves of it? And if medicolegal concerns and insufficient training render most obstetricians unsuitable for high-risk pregnancies, one must again ask what role obstetricians should have in American prenatal care.

Medical costs rise as one goes from midwife to obstetrician to maternal-fetal specialist. But do outcomes improve in relationship to the supposed expertise of the prenatal care provider? There's not a shred of credible published evidence that a given pregnancy complication will have a better outcome if it is managed by a maternal-fetal specialist instead of an obstetrician. Indeed, since maternal-fetal medicine was established as a subspecialty of obstetrics and gynecology several decades ago, our low-birthweight and prematurity rates have continued to climb. Although several explanations may be offered for this phenomenon, it is up to maternal-fetal specialists to prove their value in the current medical environment. To this end, studies comparing the outcomes of high-risk women who are managed by obstetricians versus maternal-fetal specialists should be initiated. In the event that sound research fails to show improved outcomes among pregnant women cared for by maternal-fetal specialists, we must reconsider the role of maternal-fetal specialists which places them at the top of the obstetrical food chain. On the other hand, if the data reveals significantly better outcomes among women receiving care from maternal-fetal specialists, it would bolster the need for appropriate and timely referral of complicated pregnant women to maternal-fetal specialists.

Regardless of what future studies may show, the three-tier system of prenatal care should be dismantled due to its inefficiency and the needless expense it generates. The subspecialty of maternal-fetal medicine was ostensibly created because the field of obstetrics was advancing too rapidly for one to master it over the course of a four-year residency, a notion not shared by some professors of the day. Nevertheless, a two-year (now three-year) "fellowship" was offered to those who desired special competence and expertise. As often as not, however, maternal-fetal medicine has served to shield obstetricians from medicolegal trouble by providing advice or by taking complex or undesirable patients off their hands, effectively allowing obstetricians to choose the risk level (and nuisance level) of patients which they will see. Unfortunately, as we have seen, many choose to avoid pregnant women who carry any degree of risk. Because the various diagnostic and therapeutic modalities that presently exist are largely available to both obstetricians and maternal-fetal specialists, the differences between these two groups relate more to their respective funds of knowledge and clinical experience with those modalities than anything else. If more than the standard four-year OB/GYN residency is needed to gain mastery in the specialty, it should be so mandated. What is the point of having insufficiently trained obstetricians if the only difference they offer over nurse-midwives is a larger bill? Does it not strike anyone as odd that after twelve years of training, an obstetrician should need advice on obstetric issues? On the other hand, what is the point of having so-called maternal-fetal specialists (i.e., those who have largely championed and presided over the gadgetization and medicalization of obstetrics with which we are presently saddled) if all they offer is medicolegal sanctuary for obstetricians? Whatever the results of large, prospective comparisons of obstetricians and maternal-fetal specialists, let the chips fall where they may; but in the name of more satisfactory and economical prenatal care in America, one or the other must go.

The Power of Anecdote

Unfortunately, the burden of proof has shifted from those who (despite the   **193**
data) advocate contemporary American prenatal care to those who (because
of the data) impugn it. Implied in this phenomenon is a disdain—or, at least,
a disregard—for science in favor of lesser disciplines. When facts and figures
fail to persuade, anecdote is always the final recourse. Indeed, there are few
things more powerful than a well-told story. Anecdote by its very nature is
not constrained by any obligation to be verifiable or accurate; it doesn't even
have to be true. Yet the impression it leaves can be indelible. In some re-
spects, clinical research is the accumulation of anecdotes carefully collected
under controlled circumstances—and in sufficiently large numbers. Gathered under the proper conditions, patterns emerge. But taken individually,
anecdotes are idiosyncratic and unreliable, and, not infrequently, self-serving
tools of the unscrupulous or misinformed. Because pregnancy and pregnancy-related healthcare are provocative issues, attempts to change the status quo will evoke emotions, powerful interests, and wrenching testimonials
from across social and political spectrums. When all is said and done, however, the data will speak for itself.

Clewell's Razor

Respect your Ignorance.
                                                        —William H. Clewell, M.D.

The purported benefits wrought by prenatal care have placed it beyond reproach among policymakers. Because it is "felt" to be an effective modality,
randomized clinical research—the gold standard for establishing the effectiveness of health interventions—has not been applied to prenatal care as an
entity. Instead, we presume it to be effective and act accordingly. Breakthroughs occur in obstetrics every day; but there is a difference between
breakthroughs and real progress, the latter being what we haven't had in
years. Meanwhile, the illusion of progress is sustained by a national media
which can't get enough of pop obstetrics. At the heart of this phenomenon
is the misperception that we know more than we really do.

   Clewell's Razor, as I have called it, is not a mantra for mediocrity but the
exhortation of a wise colleague to avoid unnecessary mischief while in the

service of pregnant women. When it comes to prenatal care, respecting our ignorance means:

- Acknowledging that we know less about pregnancy and its complications than we sometimes admit. It means knowing our limits.
- Not raising false hope with the illusion of technology.
- Not intimidating or comforting with the pretense of expertise.
- Not extrapolating the utility of a particular diagnostic or therapeutic modality beyond its intended application nor attributing effectiveness to any technique beyond what is implied by sound data. It also means opposing the dissemination of unsubstantiated methods of care.
- Acknowledging that good intentions do not render a particular modality more effective.

It could be argued that despite the questionable efficacy of American prenatal care, things would be even worse without it. Unfortunately, there is no way to verify or refute such claims without data. Yet it is exactly this sort of argument which has served advocates of prenatal care well; better, at least, than it has served pregnant women. Indeed, a more plausible claim is that most pregnant women do well despite the prenatal care they receive.

The legacy of American prenatal care is a perfect example of ignorance disrespected. But despite the ongoing healthcare ferment in the United States, neither reformer nor defender of the status quo have dared to assail the utility of prenatal care. The collective obstetric history of our nation is a reflection of longstanding social and economic problems. The politically expedient proposition that prenatal care can provide a simple remedy is not supported by the available evidence and reveals how poorly we understand our situation. As a result, pregnant women now find themselves not at a crossroads but on the slope of a rising prematurity rate, an incline all too well traveled by Sisyphus.

Notes

NOTES TO CHAPTER 1

1. P. G. Stubblefield. "Causes and Prevention of Premature Birth: An Overview." In *Preterm Birth: Causes, Prevention and Management.* 2nd edition. A. R. Fuchs, F. Fuchs, P. G. Stubblefield, editors. New York City: McGraw-Hill, Inc., 1993.

2. American College of Obstetricians and Gynecologists. "Commentary to 'Prenatal Care Should Be Embraced.'" *ACOG Clinical Review.* September/October 1998, p.3.

3. B. Jordan. *Birth in Four Cultures.* Montreal: Eden Press, 1983.

4. Great Britain: Parliament, Social Services Committee. *Perinatal and Neonatal Mortality, Second Report of the Social Services Committee, Volume One.* London: Her Majesty's Stationary Office, 1980, p.21.

5. R. K. Gribble, S. C. Fee, R. L. Berg. "The Value of Routine Urine Dipstick Screening for Protein at Each Prenatal Visit." *American Journal of Obstetrics and Gynecology.* 173(1995)214.

6. V. S. Kuo, G. Koumantakis, E. D. Gallery. "Proteinuria and Its Assessment in Normal and Hypertensive Pregnancy." *American Journal of Obstetrics and Gynecology.* 167(1992)723.

7. I. Lopez-Espinoza, H. Dhar, S. Humphreys, C. W. Redman. "Urinary Albumin Excretion in Pregnancy." *British Journal of Obstetrics and Gynecology.* 93 (1986)176.

8. R. W. Stettler, F. G. Cunningham. "Natural History of Chronic Proteinuria Complicating Pregnancy." *American Journal of Obstetrics and Gynecology.* 167 (1992)1219.

9. J. Sikorski, J. Wilson, S. Clement. S. Das, N. Smeeton. "A Randomized Controlled Trial Comparing Two Schedules of Antenatal Visits: The Antenatal Care Project." *British Medical Journal.* 312(1996)546.

10. I. H. Kaiser. "Reappraisals of J. Marion Sims." *American Journal of Obstetrics and Gynecology.* 132(1978)878.

11. Institute of Medicine. *Prenatal Care.* Washington, D.C.: National Academy Press, 1988, p.23.

12. M. J. Hughey. "Routine Prenatal and Gynecologic Care in Prepaid Group Practice." *Journal of the American Medical Association.* 256(1986)1775.

13. M. Haertsch, E. Campbell, R. Sanson-Fisher. "What Is Recommended for Healthy Women during Pregnancy? A Comparison of Seven Prenatal Clinical Practice Guideline Documents." *Birth.* 26(March 1999)24.

14. M. Kotelchuck. "The Adequacy of Prenatal Care Utilization Index: Its U.S. Distribution and Association with Low Birthweight." *American Journal of Public Health.* 84(1994)1486.

15. American Academy of Pediatrics and American College of Obstetricians and Gynecologists. *Guidelines for Prenatal Care.* Elk Grove Village, Ill., and Washington, D.C.: American Academy of Pediatrics and American College of Obstetricians and Gynecologists, 1988, p.87.

16. B. Blondel. "Some Characteristics of Antenatal Care in 13 European Countries." *British Journal of Obstetrics and Gynecology.* 92(1985)565.

17. Kotelchuck. "Adequacy of Prenatal Care Utilization." p.1486.

18. L. Mascarenhas, B. W. Eliot, I. Z. MacKenzie. "A Comparison of Perinatal Outcome, Antenatal and Intrapartum Care between England and Wales, and France." *British Journal of Obstetrics and Gynecology.* 99(1992)955.

19. United States Public Health Services. *Caring for Our Future: The Content of Prenatal Care.* Washington, D.C.: Department of Health and Human Services, Public Health Services, 1989, p.47.

20. M. A. Binstock, G. Wolde-Tsadik. "Alternative Prenatal Care: Impact of Reduced Visit Frequency, Focused Visits and Continuity of Care." *Journal of Reproductive Medicine.* 40(1995)507.

21. P. A. Buescher, C. Smith, J. L. Holliday, R. H. Levine. "Source of Prenatal Care and Infant Birthweight: The Case of a North Carolina County." *American Journal of Obstetrics and Gynecology.* 156(1987)204.

22. M. D. Peoples-Sheps, U. K. Hogan, N. Ng'andu. "Content of Prenatal Care during the Initial Work-up." *American Journal of Obstetrics and Gynecology.* 174 (1996)220.

23. J. C. Morrison. "Preterm Birth: A Puzzle Worth Solving." *American Journal of Obstetrics and Gynecology.* Supplement. 76(1990)55.

24. Ibid.

25. Ibid.

26. Ibid.

27. J. A. McGregor, J. I. French. "Opportunities and Obligations for Preventing Preterm Birth." *Medical Tribune.* 3(1996)13.

28. Morrison. "Preterm Birth." p.55.

29. Ibid.

30. J. A. Rogowski. "The Economics of Preterm Delivery." *Prenatal and Neonatal Medicine.* 3(1998)16.

31. Morrison. "Preterm Birth." p.55.

32. Rogowski. "The Economics of Preterm Delivery." p.16.

33. Morrison. "Preterm Birth." p.55.

34. Rogowski. "The Economics of Preterm Delivery." p.16.

35. Morrison. "Preterm Birth." p.55.

36. Rogowski. "The Economics of Preterm Delivery." p.16.

37. Children's Defense Fund. *The State of America's Children, 1992.* Washington, D.C.: Children's Defense Fund, 1992.

38. M. C. McCormick. "The Contribution of Low Birthweight to Infant

Mortality and Childhood Morbidity." *New England Journal of Medicine.* 312 (1985)82.

39. N. Paneth. "The Problem of Low Birthweight." *Future Child.* 5(1995)19.   **197**

40. B. Guyer, J. A. Martin, M. F. MacDorman, R. N. Anderson, D.M. Strobino. "Annual Summary of Vital Statistics—1996." *Pediatrics.* 100(1997)905.

41. G. J. Schieber, J. P. Poullier, L. G. Greenwald. "U.S. Health Expenditure Performance: An International Comparison and Data Update." *Health Care Financing Review.* 13(1992)15.

42. Ibid.

43. M. E. Wegman. "Infant Mortality: Some International Comparisons." *Pediatrics.* 98(1996)1020.

44. B. P. Sachs, R. C. Fretts, R. Gardner. S. Hellerstein, N. S. Wampler, P. H. Wise. "The Impact of Extreme Prematurity and Congenital Anomalies on the Interpretation of International Comparisons of Infant Mortality." *Obstetrics and Gynecology.* 85(1995)941.

45. C. Haub, M. Yanagashita. "Infant Mortality: Who's Number One?" *Population Today.* 19(1991)6.

46. J. Dobois, J. Senecal, J. R. Giraud. "Pour une Réduction de la Mortalité Perinatalé." *Journal de Gynecologic, Obstetrique et Biologie de la Reproduction* (Paris). 13(1984)491.

47. B. Branger. "Les Nouveau-nés de Poids de Naissance de 1000 G et Moins. Une Etude Régionale de 124 Cas." *Pédiatrie.* 46(1991)357.

48. K. Liu, M. Moon, M. Sulvetta, J. Chawla. "International Infant Mortality Rankings: A Look behind the Numbers." *Health Care Financing Review.* 13 (1992)105.

49. Sachs. "The Impact of Extreme Prematurity." p.941.

50. Ibid.

51. Wegman. "Infant Morality." p.1020.

52. Guyer. "Annual Summary." p.905.

53. Ibid.

54. S. G. Gabbe, J. R. Niebyl, J. L. Simpson. *Obstetrics: Normal and Problem Pregnancies.* New York: Churchill-Livingstone, 1996, p.205.

55. J. G. Wilson, F. C. Fraser. *Handbook of Teratology, Volume One.* New York: Plenum, 1977, p.75.

56. MRC Vitamin Study Research Group. "Prevention of Neural Tube Defects: Results of the Medical Research Vitamin Study." *Lancet.* 338(1991)131.

57. A. E. Czeizel, I. Dudas. "Prevention of the First Occurrence of Neural Tube Defects by Periconceptual Vitamin Supplementation." *New England Journal of Medicine.* 327(1992)1832.

58. G. K. Singh, T. J. Matthews, S. C. Clarke, T. Yannicos, B. L. Smith. *Annual Summary of Births, Marriages, Divorces and Deaths: United States, 1994.* Volume 43. Washington, D.C.: National Center for Health Statistics, 1995.

59. K. D. Peters, K. D. Kochanek, S. L. Murphy. "Deaths: Final Data for 1996." *National Vital Statistics Reports.* 47, Number 9(November 10, 1998)1.

198   60. L. Wilkins-Haug, L. Hill, L. Schmidt, G. B. Holzman, J. Schulkin. "Genetics in Obstetricians' Offices: A Survey Study." *Obstetrics and Gynecology.* 93(1999) 642.

61. Practice Management Information Corporation. *International Classification of Diseases, Ninth Revision with Clinical Modification.* Los Angeles: Practice Management Information Corporation, 1997.

62. Guyer. "Annual Summary." p.905.

63. Ibid.

64. American Academy of Pediatrics, Task Force on Infant Positioning and SIDS. "Positioning and SIDS." *Pediatrics.* 87(1992)1120.

65. Ibid.

66. R. L. Goldenberg, D. J. Rouse. "Prevention of Premature Birth." *New England Journal of Medicine.* 339(1998)313.

67. S. B. Amini, L. J. Dierker, P. M. Catalano, G. C. Ashmead, L. I. Mann. "Trends in an Obstetric Patient Population: An Eighteen-Year Study. *American Journal of Obstetrics and Gynecology.* 171(1994)1014.

68. J. C. Gersten, C. K. Mrela. *Closing the Decade: Arizona Health Status and Vital Statistics, 1980–1989.* Phoenix: Arizona Department of Health Services, 1990.

69. C. K. Mrela. *Arizona Health Status and Vital Statistics, 1995.* Phoenix: Arizona Department of Health Services, 1996.

70. J. G. Garbaciak. "Prematurity Prevention: Who Is at Risk?" *Clinics in Perinatology.* 19(1992)275.

71. R. M. Schwartz. "What Price Prematurity?" *Family Planning Perspectives.* 21(1989)170.

72. K. Prager. *Infant Mortality by Birthweight and Other Characteristics: United States, 1985 Birth Cohort.* Vital and Health Statistic Series, Volume 20, Number 24, DHHS publication number PHS 94–1852. Hyattsville, Md.: U.S. Department of Health and Human Services, Public Health Service, Centers for Disease Control and Prevention, National Center for Health Statistics, 1994.

73. Guyer. "Annual Summary." p.905.

74. R. K. Creasy. "Preventing Preterm Birth." *New England Journal of Medicine.* 325(1991)727.

75. G. R. Alexander. "Preterm Birth: Etiology, Mechanisms and Prevention." *Prenatal and Neonatal Medicine.* 3(1998)3.

76. K. Danbe, D. C. Dyson, J. A. Bamber, J. Ching. "Preterm Birth Prevention Strategies: An Analysis of Three Levels of Surveillance for Women at Risk with Singleton Gestations." *Prenatal and Neonatal Medicine.* 3(1998)157.

77. W. E. Roberts, J. C. Morrison, K. G. Perry, R. C. Floyd, B. N. McLaugh-

lin, M. D. Fox. "Risk of Preterm Delivery from Preterm Labor in High-Risk Patients." *Journal of Reproductive Medicine.* 40(1995)95.

78. American College of Obstetricians and Gynecologists. "Preterm Labor." *ACOG Technical Bulletin.* 206(1995)1.

79. M. McLean, W. A. W. Walters, R. Smith. "Prediction and Early Diagnosis of Preterm Labor: A Critical Review." *Obstetrical and Gynecological Survey.* 48(1993)209.

80. M. A. Herron, M. Katz, R. K. Creasy. "Evaluation of a Preterm Birth Prevention Program: Preliminary Report." *Obstetrics and Gynecology.* 59(1982)452.

81. E. Papiernik, J. Bouyer, J. Dreyfus, D. Collin, G. Winisdorffer, S. Guegan, et al. "Prevention of Preterm Births: A Perinatal Study in Haguenau, France." *Pediatrics.* 76(1985)154.

82. E. Muellar-Heubach, D. Reddick, B. Barnett, R. Bente. "Preterm Birth Prevention: Evaluation of a Prospective, Controlled, Randomized Trial." *American Journal of Obstetrics and Gynecology.* 160(1989)1172.

83. R. L. Goldenberg, D. O. Davis, R. L. Copper, D. K. Corliss, J. B. Andrews, A. H. Carpenter. "The Alabama Preterm Birth Prevention Project." *Obstetrics and Gynecology.* 75(1990)933.

84. F. J. McLaughlin, W. A. Altemeier, M. J. Christensen, K. B. Sherrod, M. S. Dietrich, D. T. Stern." Randomized Trial of Comprehensive Prenatal Care for Low-Income Women: Effect on Infant Birth Weight." *Pediatrics.* 89(1992)128.

85. Collaborative Group on Preterm Birth Prevention. "Multicenter Randomized, Controlled Trial of a Preterm Birth Prevention Program." *American Journal of Obstetrics and Gynecology.* 169(1993)352.

86. C. J. Hobel, M. G. Ross, R. L. Bemis, J. R. Bragonier, S. Nessim, M. Sandhu, et al. "The West Los Angeles Preterm Birth Prevention Project: I. Program Impact on High-Risk Women. *American Journal of Obstetrics and Gynecology.* 170(1994)54.

87. R. L. Bryce, F. J. Stanley, B. J. Garner. "Randomized, Controlled Trial of Antenatal Social Support to Prevent Preterm Birth." *British Journal of Obstetrics and Gynecology.* 98(1991)1001.

88. D. L. Olds, C. R. Henderson, R. Tatelbaum, R. Chamberlin. "Improving the Delivery of Prenatal Care and Outcomes of Pregnancy: A Randomized Trial of Nurse Home Visitation." *Pediatrics.* 77(1986)16.

89. D. M. Main, S. G. Gabbe, D. K. Richardson, S. Strong. "Can Preterm Deliveries Be Prevented?" *American Journal of Obstetrics and Gynecology.* 151(1985) 892.

90. D. M. Main, D. K. Richardson, C. B. Hadley, S. G. Gabbe. "Controlled Trial of a Preterm Labor Detection Program: Efficacy and Costs." *Obstetrics and Gynecology.* 74(1989)873.

91. B. Spencer, H. Thomas, J. Morris. "A Randomized, Controlled Trial of the

Provision of a Social Support Service during Pregnancy: The South Manchester Family Worker Project." *British Journal of Obstetrics and Gynecology.* 96(1989) 281.

92. H. C. Heins, N. W. Nance, B. J. McCarthy, C. M. Efird. "A Randomized Trial of Nurse-Midwifery Prenatal Care to Reduce Low Birth Weight." *Obstetrics and Gynecology.* 75(1990)341.

93. A. V. Graham, S. H. Frank, S. J. Zyzanski, G. C. Kitson, K. G. Reeb. "A Clinical Trial to Reduce the Rate of Low Birth Weight in an Inner-City Black Population." *Family Medicine.* 24(1992)439.

94. J. Villar, U. Farnot, F. Barros, C. Victoria, A. Langer, J. M. Belizan. "A Randomized Trial of Psychosocial Support during High-Risk Pregnancies: The Latin American Network for Perinatal and Reproductive Research." *New England Journal of Medicine.* 327(1992)1266.

95. Herron. "A Preterm Birth Prevention Program." p.452.

96. Papiernik. "Prevention of Preterm Birth." p.154.

97. C. Holzman, N. Paneth. "Preterm Birth: From Prediction to Prevention." *American Journal of Public Health.* 88(1998)183.

98. P. J. Meis, J. M. Ernest, M. L. Moore, R. Michielutte, P. C. Sharp, P. A. Buescher. "Regional Program for Prevention of Premature Birth in Northwestern North Carolina." *American Journal of Obstetrics and Gynecology.* 157(1987)550.

99. Gersten. "Closing the Decade."

100. Peoples-Sheps. "Content of Prenatal Care." p.220.

101. N. T. Eastman. "Prematurity from the Viewpoint of the Obstetrician." *American Practitioner.* 1(1947)343.

102. K. Byrne. "Prenatal Program Aims to Head-Off Expensive Emergency Care." *Arizona Republic.* December 26, 1995, p.B-6.

103. Institute of Medicine. *Preventing Low Birthweight.* Washington, D.C.: National Academy Press, 1985, p.147.

104. C. Holzman, N. Paneth, R. Fisher, The Prematurity Prevention Group. "Rethinking the Concept of Risk Factors for Preterm Delivery: Antecedents, Markers and Mediators." *Prenatal and Neonatal Medicine.* 3(1998)47.

105. Alexander. "Preterm Birth." p.3.

106. Jordan. "Birth in Four Cultures." p.74.

107. J. H. Kennell, M. H. Klaus. "The Perinatal Paradigm: Is It Time for a Change?" *Current Controversies in Perinatal Care.* 4(1988)801.

108. J. Mitford. *The American Way of Birth.* New York: Penguin Books, 1992.

NOTES TO CHAPTER 2

1. March of Dimes. *The Promise of Science: March of Dimes Research Annual Report—1998.* White Plains, N.Y.: March of Dimes Birth Defects Foundation, 1998, p.9.

200

2. H. F. Sandmire. "Whither Tocolysis?" *Birth.* 23(1996)38.

3. N. J. Eastman. "*Obstetrics and Gynecology.*" In *Seventy-Five Years of Medical Progress: 1878–1953.* L. H. Bauer, editor. Philadelphia: Lea and Febiger, **201** 1954, p.89.

4. J. W. Ballantyne. "A Plea for a Pro-Maternity Hospital." *British Medical Journal.* Number 2101 (April 6, 1901)813.

5. J. W. Ballantyne. "Visits to the Wards of the Pro-Maternity Hospital: A Vision of the Twentieth Century." *American Journal of Obstetrics.* 43(1901)593.

6. H. Speert. *Obstetrics and Gynecology in America, A History.* Baltimore: Waverly Press, 1980, p.142.

7. Ibid.

8. C. E. Heaton. "Fifty Years of Progress in Obstetrics and Gynecology." *New York State Journal of Medicine.* 51(1951)83.

9. Speert. *Obstetrics and Gynecology in America.* p.142.

10. R. W. Wertz, D. C. Wertz. *Lying-In: A History of Childbirth in America.* New York: Free Press, 1978.

11. Ibid.

12. *Illinois Medical Journal.* 39, Number 143 (February 1921).

13. M. Sheppard, H. M. Towner. *United States Senate Bill Number 3259.* 1919.

14. Speert. *Obstetrics and Gynecology in America.* p.142.

15. J. L. Huntington. "Relation of the Hospital to the Hygiene of Pregnancy." *Boston Medical and Surgical Journal.* 169(1913)763.

16. Institute of Medicine. *Preventing Low Birthweight.* Washington, D.C.: National Academy Press, 1985.

17. J. Huntington, F. A. Connell. "For Every Dollar Spent—The Cost-Savings Argument for Prenatal Care." *New England Journal of Medicine.* 331(1994)1303.

18. M. C. McCormick, D. K. Richardson. "Prevention and Intervention Research: Economic Issues." *Prenatal and Neonatal Medicine.* 3(1998)173.

19. W. J. Smith, C. C. Blackmore. "Economic Analysis in Obstetrics and Gynecology: A Methodologic Evaluation of the Literature." *Obstetrics and Gynecology.* 91(1998)472.

20. Institute of Medicine. "Prenatal Care and Low Birthweight: Effects on Health Care Expenditures." *Preventing Low Birthweight.* Washington, D.C.: National Academy Press, 1994, p.212.

21. K. Fiscella. "Does Prenatal Care Improve Birth Outcomes? A Critical Review." *Obstetrics and Gynecology.* 85(1995)468.

22. Huntington. "For Every Dollar Spent." p.1303.

23. J. O. Mason. "Reducing Infant Mortality in the United States through 'Healthy Start.'" *Public Health Reports.* 106(1991)479.

24. Ibid.

25. D. Morgan. "U.S. Says Infant Mortality Report Wasn't Squelched." *Reuters.* November 12, 1997.

26. Ibid.

27. P. H. Wise. "What You Measure Is What You Get: Prenatal Care and
202 Women's Health." *American Journal of Public Health.* 84(1994)1374.

28. National Center for Health Statistics. *Health, United States, 1993.* DHHS
publication number 94-1232. Hyattsville, Md.: Public Health Service, 1984.

29. J. Gates-Williams, M. N. Jackson, V. Jenkins-Monroe, L. R. Williams.
"Cross-Cultural Medicine a Decade Later: The Business of Preventing African-
American Infant Mortality." *Western Journal of Medicine.* 157(1992)350.

30. Fiscella. "Does Prenatal Care Improve Birth Outcomes?" p.468.

31. Institute of Medicine. "Infant Death: An Analysis by Maternal Risk and
Health Care." In *Contrasts in Healthcare.* Volume 1. D. M. Kessner, editor. Washington, D.C.: National Academy of Sciences, 1973.

32. M. H. Hall. "Commentary: What Are the Benefits of Prenatal Care in Uncomplicated Pregnancy?" *Birth.* 18(1991)151.

33. D. A. Grimes. "How Can We Translate Good Science into Good Perinatal
Care?" *Birth.* 13(1986)83.

34. G. Lindmark, S. Cnattingius. "The Scientific Basis of Antenatal Care: Report from a State of the Art Conference." *Acta Obstetrics and Gynecology of Scandinavia.* 70(1991)105.

35. A. L. Cochrane. "1931–1971: A Critical Review with Particular Reference
to the Medical Profession." In *Medicines for the Year 2000.* London: Office of
Health Economics, 1979.

36. I. Chalmers. "Evaluating the Effects of Care during Pregnancy and Childbirth." In I. Chalmers, M. Enkin, M. J. N. C. Keirse, editors. *Effective Care in
Pregnancy and Childbirth.* Oxford: Oxford University Press, 1989.

37. J. E. Tyson, J. A. Furzan, J. S. Reisch, S. G. Mize. "An Evaluation of the
Quality of Therapeutic Studies in Perinatal Medicine." *Obstetrics and Gynecology.*
62(1983)99.

38. Chalmers. "Evaluating the Effects of Care." p.3.

39. L. Klein, R. L. Goldenberg. "Prenatal Care and Its Effect on Preterm Birth
and Low Birthweight." In *New Perspectives on Prenatal Care.* I. R. Merkatz, J. E.
Thompson, editors. New York: Elsevier, 1993, p.501.

40. Institute of Medicine. *Preventing Low Birthweight.* Washington, D.C.: National Academy Press, 1985, p.147.

41. A. Fink, E. M. Yano, D. Goya. "Prenatal Programs: What the Literature Reveals." *Obstetrics and Gynecology.* 80(1992)867.

42. S. H. Kane. "Significance of Prenatal Care." *Obstetrics and Gynecology.* 24
(1964)66.

43. T. Raine, S. Powell, M. A. Krohn. "The Risk of Repeating Low Birth Weight
and the Role of Prenatal Care." *Obstetrics and Gynecology.* 84(1994)485.

44. R. Mittendorf, M. Herschel, M. A. Williams, J. U. Hibbard, A. H. Moawad,

K. S. Lee. "Reducing the Frequency of Low Birthweight in the United States." *Obstetrics and Gynecology.* 83(1994)1056.

45. M. J. Tucker, R. L. Goldenberg, R. O. Davis, R. L. Copper, C. L. Winkler, J. C. Hauth. "Etiologies of Preterm Birth in an Indigent Population: Is Prevention a Logical Expectation?" *Obstetrics and Gynecology.* 77(1991)343.

46. W. Silverman. "The Optimistic Bias Favoring Medical Action." *Controlled Clinical Trials.* 12(1991)557.

47. R. J. Apfel, S. M. Fisher. *To Do Harm: DES and the Dilemma of Modern Medicine.* New Haven: Yale University Press, 1984.

48. L. S. Bakketeig, H. J. Hoffman, E. E. Harley. "The Tendency to Repeat Gestational Age and Birth Weight in Successive Births." *American Journal of Obstetrics and Gynecology.* 135(1979)1080.

49. P. Lazar, S. Gueguen. "Multicentered Controlled Trial of Cervical Cerclage in Women at Moderate Risk of Preterm Delivery." *British Journal of Obstetrics and Gynecology.* 91(1984)731.

50. R. W. Rush. "A Randomized, Controlled Trial of Cervical Cerclage in Women at High Risk of Spontaneous Preterm Delivery." *British Journal of Obstetrics and Gynecology.* 91(1984)724.

51. MRC/RCOG Working Party on Cervical Cerclage. "Final Report of the Medical Research Council/Royal College of Obstetricians and Gynecologists Multicentre Randomized Trial of Cervical Cerclage." *British Journal of Obstetrics and Gynecology.* 100(1993)516.

52. Rush. "A Randomized Trial of Cervical Cerclage." p.724.

53. Ibid.

54. Ibid.

55. D. M. Main, E. K. Main. "Management of Preterm Labor and Delivery." *Obstetrics: Normal and Problem Pregnancies.* In. S. G. Gabbe, J. R. Niebyl, J. L. Simpson, editors. New York: Churchill Livingstone, 1986, p. 689.

56. M. J. N. C. Keirse. "Beta-Mimetic Drugs in the Prophylaxis of Preterm Labour: Extent and Rationale of Their Use." *British Journal of Obstetrics and Gynecology.* 91(1984)431.

57. G. A. Macones, M. Berlin, J. A. Berlin. "Efficacy of Oral Beta-Agonist Maintenance Therapy in Preterm Labor: A Meta-Analysis. *Obstetrics and Gynecology.* 85(1995)313.

58. K. D. Wenstrom, C. P. Weiner, D. Merrill, J. Niebyl. "A Placebo-Controlled, Randomized Trial of the Terbutaline Pump for Prevention of Preterm Delivery." *American Journal of Perinatology.* 14(1997)87.

59. D. A. Guinn, A. R. Goepfert, J. Owen, K. D. Wenstrom, J. C. Hauth. "Terbutaline Pump Maintenance Therapy for Prevention of Preterm Delivery: A Double-Blind Trial." *American Journal of Obstetrics and Gynecology.* 179(1998) 874.

60. American College of Obstetricians and Gynecologists. "Preterm Labor." *ACOG Technical Bulletin.* 206(1995).

204   61. S. L. Nightingale. "From the Food and Drug Administration." *Journal of the American Medical Association.* 279(1998)9.

62. M. McClean, W. A. W. Walters, R. Smith. "Prediction and Early Diagnosis of Preterm Labor: A Critical Review." *Obstetrical and Gynecological Review.* 48 (1993)209.

63. D. A. Grimes, K. F. Schulz. "Randomized, Controlled Trials of Home Uterine Activity Monitoring: A Review and Critique." *Obstetrics and Gynecology.* 79 (1992)164.

64. The Collaborative Home Uterine Monitoring Study (CHUMS) Group. "A Multicenter Randomized, Controlled Trial of Home Uterine Monitoring: Active versus Sham Device." *American Journal of Obstetrics and Gynecology.* 173(1995) 1120.

65. United States Preventive Services Task Force. "Home Uterine Activity Monitoring for Preterm Labor: Policy Statement." *Journal of the American Medical Association.* 270(1993)369.

66. ACOG Technical Bulletin. 206(June 1995)3.

67. R. L. Goldenberg. "Unresolved Controversies: Home Uterine Activity Monitoring." *Birth.* 19(1992)164.

68. H. J. Finberg. "Routine Ultrasound Screening in Pregnancy: Tough Questions." *Radiology Today.* 10(1993)3.

69. J. P. Crane, M. L. LeFevre, R. C. Winborn, et al. "A Randomized Trial of Prenatal Ultrasonographic Screening: Impact on the Detection, Management and Outcome of Anomalous Fetuses." *American Journal of Obstetrics and Gynecology.* 171(1994)392.

70. B. Baker. "Lawsuits Rising for Missed Anomaly on Ultrasound." *OB/GYN News.* 31(1996)5.

71. D. A. Nagey. "The Content of Prenatal Care." *Obstetrics and Gynecology.* 74 (1989)516.

72. E. Hemminki, B. Starfield. "Routine Administration of Iron and Vitamins during Pregnancy: Review of Controlled Clinical Trials." *British Journal of Obstetrics and Gynecology.* 85(1978)404.

73. R. Rubin. "The Baby or the Drug?" *U.S. News and World Report.* March 27, 1995, p.59.

74. Ibid.

75. C. P. Crowley, I. Chalmers, M. J. N. C. Keirse. "The Effects of Corticosteroid Administration before Preterm Delivery: An Overview of the Evidence from Controlled Trials." *British Journal of Obstetrics and Gynecology.* 97(1990)11.

76. National Institute of Health. "Effect of Corticosteroids for Fetal Maturation on Perinatal Outcome." *NIH Consensus Statement.* 12(1994)1.

77. D. A. Grimes. "Introducing Evidence-Based Medicine into a Department of *Obstetrics and Gynecology.*" *Obstetrics and Gynecology.* 86(1995)451.

78. W. J. Hueston. "Preterm Contractions in Community Settings: Treatment of Preterm Contractions." *Obstetrics and Gynecology.* 92(1998)38.

79. C. J. Lockwood, A. E. Senyei, M. R. Dische. "Fetal Fibronectin in Cervical and Vaginal Secretions Defines a Patient Population at High Risk for Preterm Delivery." *New England Journal of Medicine.* 325(1991)669.

80. C. J. Lockwood, R. Wein, R. Lapinski, R. Alvarez, R. Berkowitz. "Fetal Fibronectin Predicts Preterm Deliveries in Asymptomatic Patients." *American Journal of Obstetrics and Gynecology.* 168(1993)311.

81. A. Revah, M. E. Hannah, A. K. Sue-A-Quan. "Fetal Fibronectin as a Predictor of Preterm Birth: An Overview." *American Journal of Perinatology.* 15 (1998)613.

82. P. W. Huber. *Galileo's Revenge: Junk Science in the Courtroom.* New York: Basic Books, 1991.

83. E. F. Funai. "Obstetrics and Gynecology in 1996: Marking the Progress toward Evidence-Based Medicine by Classifying Studies Based on Methodology." *Obstetrics and Gynecology.* 90(1997)1020.

NOTES TO CHAPTER 3

1. J. G. Jollis, E. D. Peterson, E. R. DeLong, et al. "The Relation between the Volume of Coronary Angioplasty Procedures at Hospitals Treating Medicare Beneficiaries and Short-Term Mortality." *New England Journal of Medicine.* 331 (1994)1625.

2. S. L. Powell, V. L. Holt, D. E. Hickok, T. Easterling, F. A. Connell. "Recent Changes in Delivery Site of Low-Birth-Weight Infants in Washington: Impact on Birth Weight-Specific Mortality." *American Journal of Obstetrics and Gynecology.* 173(1995)1585.

3. L. S. Bakketeig, H. J. Hoffman, P. M. Sternthal. "Obstetric Service and Perinatal Mortality in Norway." *Acta Obstetrics and Gynecology of Scandinavia.* Supplement. 77(1978)3.

4. N. Paneth, J. L. Kiely, S. Wallenstein, M. Marcus, J. Pakter, M. Susser. "Newborn Intensive Care and Neonatal Mortality in Low Birth-Weight Infants." *New England Journal of Medicine.* 307(1982)149.

5. Powell. "Recent Changes in Delivery Site." p.1585.

6. R. A. Rosenblatt, J. A. Mayfield, L. G. Hart, L. M. Baldwin. "Outcomes of Regionalized Perinatal Care in Washington State." *Western Journal of Medicine.* 149(1988)98.

7. L. O. Lubchenco, L. J. Butterfield, V. Delaney-Black, E. Goldson, B. L. Koops, D. C. Lazotte. "Outcome of Very-Low-Birth-Weight Infants: Does

Antepartum versus Neonatal Referral Have a Better Impact on Mortality, Morbidity or Long-Term Outcome?" *American Journal of Obstetrics and Gynecology.* 160 (1989)539.

206

8. R. J. Ozminkowski, P. M. Wortman, D. W. Roloff. "Inborn/Outborn Status and Neonatal Survival: A Meta-Analysis of Non-Randomized Studies." *Statistics in Medicine.* 7(1988)1207.

9. W. Kitchen, G. Ford, A. Orgill, et al. "Outcome of Extremely Low Birth-Weight Infants in Relation to the Hospital of Birth." *Australian and New Zealand Journal of Obstetrics and Gynecology.* 24(1984)1.

10. D. Gagnon, S. Allison-Cooke, R. M. Schwartz. "Perinatal Care: The Threat of Deregionalization." *Pediatric Annals.* 17(1988)447.

11. P. G. Tomich, C. L. Anderson. "Analysis of a Maternal Transport Service within a Perinatal Region." *American Journal of Perinatology.* 7(1990)13.

12. J. P. Elliott, T. L. Sipp, K. T. Balazs. "Maternal Transport of Patients with Advanced Cervical Dilatation—To Fly or Not to Fly?" *Obstetrics and Gynecology.* 79(1992)380.

13. Rosenblatt. "Outcomes of Regionalized Perinatal Care." p.98.

14. J. A. Mayfield, R. A. Rosenblatt, L. M. Baldwin, J. Chu, J. P. LoGerfo. "The Relation of Obstetrical Volume and Nursery Level to Perinatal Mortality." *American Journal of Public Health.* 80(1990)819.

15. S. Borker, C. Rudolph, T. Tsuruki, M. Williams. "Interhospital Referral of High-Risk Newborns in a Rural Regional Perinatal Program." *Journal of Perinatology.* 10(1990)156.

16. Powell. "Recent Changes in Delivery Site." p.1585.

17. R. Keller. "Dealing with Geographic Variations in Medical Care among Small Areas: The Experience of the Maine Medical Assessment Program's Orthopaedic Study Group." *Journal of Bone and Joint Surgery.* (October 1990) 1286.

18. R. D. Lamm. "Healthcare Heresies." *Healthcare Forum Journal.* (September/October 1994)45.

19. S. R. Eastaugh. *Health Economics: Efficiency, Quality and Equity.* Westport, Conn.: Greenwood Publishing, 1992.

20. A. David. "Unsound Sonograms?" *Parenting.* (April 1995)21.

21. C. Craft. "From a Woman's Point of View." *Today's Health Care.* December 1994, p.4.

22. Eastaugh. "Health Economics." p. 71.

23. Z. Dyckman. *A Study of Physician Fees.* Staff Report, Council on Wage and Price Stability, Executive Office of the President. Washington, D.C.: U.S. Government Printing Office, March 1978.

24. Institute of Medicine. *Medicare-Medicaid Reimbursement Policies, Part 3, Volume 3.* Washington, D.C.: National Academy of Sciences, 1976.

25. J. Newhouse, C. Phelps. "New Estimates of Price and Income Elasticities of

Medical Care Services." In *The Role of Health Insurance in the Health Services Sector.* R. Rosett, editor. New York: Watson Academic, 1976, p.216.

26. J. Holahan, W. Scanlon. *Physician Pricing in California: Price Controls,* **207** *Physician Fees, and Physician Incomes from Medicare and Medicaid.* Washington, D.C.: U.S. Department of Health, Education, and Welfare, Health Care Financing Administration, 1979.

27. Institute of Medicine. *The Effect of Medical Professional Liability on the Delivery of Obstetric Care.* Washington, D.C.: National Academy Press, 1989.

28. D. I. Allen, J. M. Kamradt. "Relationship of Infant Mortality to Availability of Obstetric Care in Indiana." *Journal of Family Practice.* 33(1991)609.

29. J. Yankowitz, D. M. Howser, J. W. Ely. "A Statewide Pattern of Access to Prenatal Care." *American Journal of Obstetrics and Gynecology.* Number 1, Part 2(1996)339.

30. S. A. Dobie, L. G. Hart, M. Fordyce, R. A. Rosenblatt. "Do Women Choose Their Obstetric Providers Based on Risks at Entry into Prenatal Care? A Study of Women in Washington State." *Obstetrics and Gynecology.* 84(1994)557.

31. E. R. Declercq. "Midwifery Care and Medical Complications: The Role of Risk Screening." *Birth.* 2(June 1995)68.

32. J. C. Gersten, C. K. Mrela. *Closing the Decade: Arizona Health Status and Vital Statistics, 1980–1989.* Phoenix: Arizona Department of Health Services, 1990.

33. C. K. Mrela. *Arizona Health Status and Vital Statistics, 1995.* Phoenix: Arizona Department of Health Services, 1996.

34. Gersten. "Closing the Decade." p.43.

35. Mrela. "Arizona Health Status." p.256.

36. Gersten. "Closing the Decade." p.28.

37. B. Guyer. "Medicaid and Prenatal Care: Necessary but Not Sufficient." *Journal of the American Medical Association.* 264(1990)2264.

38. Institute of Medicine. *Preventing Low Birthweight.* Washington, D.C.: National Academic Press, 1985.

39. P. Braveman, T. Bennett, C. Lewis, S. Egerter, J. Showstack. "Access to Perinatal Care Following Major Medicaid Eligibility Expansions." *Journal of the American Medical Association.* 269(1993)1285.

40. J. M. Piper, W. A. Ray, M. R. Griffin. "Effects of Medicaid Eligibility Expansion on Prenatal Care and Pregnancy Outcome in Tennessee." *Journal of the American Medical Association.* 264(1990)2219.

41. J. S. Haas, I. S. Udvarhely, C. N. Morris, A. M. Epstein. "The Effect of Providing Health Coverage to Poor, Uninsured Pregnant Women in Massachusetts." *Journal of the American Medical Association.* 269(1993)87.

42. L. M. Baldwin, E. H. Larson, F. A. Connell, et al. "The Effect of Expanding Medicaid Prenatal Services on Birth Outcomes." *American Journal of Public Health.* 88(1998)1623.

43. Ibid.

44. C. C. Korenbrot, A. Gill, Z. Clayson, E. Patterson. "Evaluation of California's Statewide Implementation of Enhanced Perinatal Services as Medicaid Benefits." *Public Health Reports.* 110(March/April 1995)125.

45. Guyer. "Medicaid and Prenatal Care." p.2264.

46. J. W. Krieger, F. A. Connell, J. P. LoGerfo. "Medicaid Prenatal Care: A Comparison of Use and Outcomes in Fee-For-Service and Managed Care." *American Journal of Public Health.* 82(1992)185.

47. W. Parchment, G. Weiss, M. R. Passannante. "Is the Lack of Health Insurance the Major Barrier to Early Prenatal Care at an Inner-City Hospital?" *Women's Health Issues.* 6(March/April 1996)97.

48. M. L. Poland, J. Ager, J. Olson. "Barriers to Receiving Adequate Prenatal Care." *American Journal of Obstetrics and Gynecology.* 157(1987)297.

49. J. P. Kugler, F. A. Connell, C. E. Henley. "An Evaluation of Prenatal Care Utilization in a Military Health Care Setting." *Military Medicine.* 155(1990)33.

50. J. V. Quick, M. Greenlick, K. Rogmann, et al. "Perinatal Care and Pregnancy Outcome in an HMO and General Population: A Multivariate Cohort Analysis." *American Journal of Public Health.* 71(1981)381.

51. E. Friedman. *The Aloha Way: Healthcare Structure and Finance in Hawaii.* Honolulu: Hawaii Medical Service Association, 1993.

52. U.S. General Accounting Office. *Healthcare in Hawaii: Implications for National Reform.* Washington, D.C.: U.S. General Accounting Office, 1994 (Document GAO/HEHS—94-68).

53. M. P. Laken, J. Ager. "Using Incentives to Increase Participation in Prenatal Care." *Obstetrics and Gynecology.* 85(1995)326.

54. P. H. Wise. "Confronting Racial Disparities in Infant Mortality: Reconciling Science and Politics." In *Racial Differences in Preterm Delivery: Developing a New Research Paradigm.* Oxford: Oxford University Press, 1993, p.7.

55. F. Mullan, M. L. Rivo, R. M. Politzer. "Doctors, Dollars and Determination: Making Physician Work-Force Policy." *Health Affairs.* Supplement (1993) 138.

56. J. E. Wennberg, D. C. Goodman, R. F. Nease, R. B. Keller. "Finding Equilibrium in U.S. Physician Supply." *Health Affairs.* (Summer 1993)89.

57. Ibid.

58. R. Kronick. "The Marketplace in Health Care Reform." *New England Journal of Medicine.* 328(1993)148.

59. J. K. Inglehart. "Health Policy Report: Healthcare Reform and Medical Education." *New England Journal of Medicine.* 330(1994)1167.

60. R. W. Hale. "The Obstetrician and Gynecologist: Primary Care Physician or Specialist?" *American Journal of Obstetrics and Gynecology.* 172(1995)1181.

61. Council on Graduate Medical Education. *Improving Access to Health Care*

through Physician Workforce Reform: Directions for the 21st Century. Washington, D.C.: U.S. Department of Health and Human Services, 1992.

62. Inglehart. "Health Policy Report." p.1167.

63. C. Morain. "Will Move to Primary Care Spell Disaster for Gynecologic Laparoscopic Surgery?" *OB/GYN and Endoscopy News.* 3(1995)1.

64. C. Kilgore. "OB/GYN's Don't Make the Primary Care Cut." *OB/GYN News.* 31(May 1, 1996)4.

65. S. Leader, P. J. Perales. "Provision of Primary—Preventive Health Care Services by Obstetrician-Gynecologists." *Obstetrics and Gynecology.* 85(1995)391.

66. R. Ranney, D. Holzwarth, R. Thornton, M. MacNeal. "The Practice of Gynecology and Obstetrics, An Analysis." *Obstetrics and Gynecology.* 47(1976) 725.

67. R. Ranney. "Shadow or Lights?" *American Journal of Obstetrics and Gynecology.* 125(1976)283.

68. Hale. "The Obstetrician and Gynecologist." p.1181.

69. M. Kuffel. "Reactions of Residency Directors to Primary Care Requirements in Obstetrics and Gynecology Training." *Obstetrics and Gynecology.* 91 (1998)145.

70. K. Podratz. "Gynecologic Surgery: An Imperiled Ballet." *American Journal of Obstetrics and Gynecology.* 178(1998)1229.

71. Committee on Health Care for Underserved Women, American College of Obstetricians and Gynecologists. *Obstetric and Gynecologic Services for Indigent Women: Issues Raised by an ACOG Survey.* Washington, D.C.: American College of Obstetricians and Gynecologists, 1988.

72. M. L. Rivo, J. W. Saultz, S. A. Wartman, T. G. DeWitt. "Defining the Generalist Physician's Training." *Journal of the American Medical Association.* 271 (1994)1499.

73. W. G. Goldberg, M. C. Tomalanovich. "Domestic Violence in the Emergency Department." *Journal of the American Medical Association.* 251(1984) 3259.

74. S. V. McLeer, R. A. H. Anwar, S. Herman, K. Maquiling. "Education Is Not Enough: A System's Failure in Protecting Battered Women." *Annals of Emergency Medicine.* 18(1989)651.

75. L. R. Chambliss, C. Bay, R. F. Jones. "Domestic Violence: An Educational Imperative?" *American Journal of Obstetrics and Gynecology.* 172(1995)1035.

76. D. L. Horan, J. Chapin, L. Klein, L. A. Schmidt, J. Schulkin. "Domestic Violence Screening Practices of Obstetrician-Gynecologists." *Obstetrics and Gynecology.* 92(1998)785.

77. Wennberg. "Finding Equilibrium in U.S. Physician Supply." p.89.

78. W. Droegemueller. "Time to Discard the Cookie Cutter." *American Journal of Obstetrics and Gynecology.* 180(1999)889.

NOTES TO CHAPTER 4

210

1. A. Cunningham. "The Rebirth of Midwifery." *Parenting.* April 1995, p.98.

2. D. A. Grimes, W. Cates. "The Impact of State Maternal Mortality Study Committees on Maternal Deaths in the United States." *American Journal of Public Health.* 67(1977)830.

3. M. L. May, D. B. Stengel. "Who Sues Their Doctors? How Patients Handle Medical Grievances." *Law and Society Review.* 24(1990)105.

4. Grimes. "The Impact of State Maternal Mortality Study." p.830.

5. D. Schipani. "The New Mom's Hospital Stay: Is It Over Too Soon?" *Child.* 6(1991)60.

6. OB/GYN Management. "OB/GYNs' Incomes Rebound Modestly." *OB/GYN Management.* January 1995, p.10.

7. D. Oakley, M. E. Murray, T. Murtland. "Comparisons of Maternity Care by Obstetricians and Certified Nurse-Midwives." *Obstetrics and Gynecology.* 88(1996) 823.

8. L. M. Walker. "OBG's Struggle to Keep Costs from Rising Too Fast." *Medical Economics—Obstetrics/Gynecology Edition.* November 1994, p.18.

9. K. Foley, L. A. Lynch. "Vital Signs." *OB/GYN News.* 34(June 15, 1999)1.

10. Committee on Health Care for Underserved Women, American College of Obstetricians and Gynecologists. *Obstetric and Gynecologic Services for Indigent Women: Issues Raised by an ACOG Survey.* Washington, D.C.: American College of Obstetricians and Gynecologists, 1988.

11. B. M. Aved, M. M. Irwin, L. S. Cummings, N. Findeisen. "Barriers to Prenatal Care for Low-Income Women." *Western Journal of Medicine.* 158(1993) 493.

12. Ibid.

13. T. R. Moore, R. T. Andrews. "Differential Litigiousness among Obstetric Patients by Payor Source." *American Journal of Obstetrics and Gynecology.* 164, Number 1, Part 2(1991)327.

14. H. R. Burstin, W. G. Johnson, S. R. Lipsitz, T. A. Brennan. "Do the Poor Sue More? A Case-Control Study of Malpractice Claims and Socioeconomic Status." *Journal of the American Medical Association.* 270(1993)1697.

15. C. Newhart, S. Teran, B. M. Aved, A. Gemmil, W. B. Harer, A. Fink. *Obstetrical Malpractice Suits among Medi-Cal Patients in Relation to the General OB Patient Population in California.* Sacramento: Sierra Health Foundation, 1990.

16. M. G. Mussman, L. Zawistowich, C. S. Weisman, F. E. Malitz, L. L. Morlock. "Medical Malpractice Claims Filed by Medicaid and Non-Medicaid Recipients in Maryland." *Journal of the American Medical Association.* 265(1991)2992.

17. United States Congress, Office of Technology Assessment. *Nurse-Practitioners, Physician Assistants and Certified Nurse-Midwives: A Policy Analysis.* Washington, D.C.: U.S. Government Printing Office, 1986.

18. Institute of Medicine. *Preventing Low Birthweight*. Washington, D.C.: National Academy Press, 1985.

19. C. Slome, H. Wetherbee, M. Daly, K. Christensen, M. Meglen, H. Thiede. **211** "Effectiveness of Certified Nurse-Midwives: A Prospective Evaluation Study." *American Journal of Obstetrics and Gynecology*. 124(1976)177.

20. G. Young. "Rethinking Antenatal Care." *Practitioner*. 236(1992)293.

21. G. B. Hickson, E. W. Clayton, P. B. Githens, F. A. Sloan. "Factors That Prompted Families to File Medical Malpractice Claims Following Perinatal Injuries." *Journal of the American Medical Association*. 267(1992)1359.

22. May. "Who Sues Their Doctors?" p.105.

23. Hickson. "Factors That Prompted Families." p.1359.

24. E. Lehrman. "Nurse-Midwifery Practice: A Descriptive Study of Prenatal Care." *Journal of Nurse Midwifery*. 26(1981)1.

25. National Center for Health Statistics. *Office Visits by Women: The National Ambulatory Medical Care Survey*. Vital and Health Statistics. Series 13, Number 45. DHHS publication number (PHS) 80-1976. Washington, D.C.: Public Health Service, March 1980.

26. Slome. "Effectiveness of Certified Nurse-Midwives." p.177.

27. H. Blanchette. "Comparison of Obstetric Outcome of a Primary-Care Access Clinic Staffed by Certified Nurse-Midwives and a Private Practice Group of Obstetricians in the Same Community." *American Journal of Obstetrics and Gynecology*. 172(1995)1864.

28. Ibid.

29. Ibid.

30. L. Mascarenhas, B. W. Eliot, I. Z. MacKenzie. "A Comparison of Perinatal Outcome, Antenatal and Intrapartum Care between England and Wales, and France." *British Journal of Obstetrics and Gynecology*. 99(1992)955.

31. L. D. Platt, D. N. Angelina, E. J. Quilligan. "Nurse-Midwifery in a Large Teaching Hospital." *Obstetrics and Gynecology*. 66(1985)816.

32. D. B. Haire, C. C. Elsberry. "Maternity Care and Outcome in a High Risk Service: The North Central Bronx Hospital Experience." *Birth*. 18(1991)33.

33. L. Schimmel, P. Hogan, B. Boehler, M. Difelice, A Cooney. "The Yolo County Midwifery Service: A Descriptive Study of 496 Singleton Birth Outcomes, 1990." *Journal of Nurse-Midwifery*. 37(1992)398.

34. B. S. Levy, F. S. Wilkinson, W. M. Marin. "Reducing Neonatal Mortality Rate with Nurse-Midwives." *American Journal of Obstetrics and Gynecology*. 109 (1971)50.

35. R. J. Mann. "San Francisco General Hospital Nurse-Midwifery Practice: The First Thousand Births." *American Journal of Obstetrics and Gynecology*. 140 (1981)676.

36. S. L. Piechnik, M. A. Corbett. "Reducing Low Birth Weight among Socioeconomically High-Risk Adolescent Pregnancies: Successful Intervention with

Certified Nurse-Midwife Managed Care and a Multidisciplinary Team." *Journal of Nurse-Midwifery.* 30(1985)88.

212

37. Slome. "Effectiveness of Certified Nurse-Midwives." p.177.

38. Blanchette. "Comparisons of Obstetric Outcome." p.1864.

39. J. E. Burnett. "A Physician-Sponsored Community Nurse-Midwife Program." *Obstetrics and Gynecology.* 40(1972)719.

40. J. C. Record, H. R. Cohen. "The Introduction of Midwifery in a Prepaid Group Practice." *American Journal of Public Health.* 62(1972)354.

41. Mascarenhas. "A Comparison of Perinatal Outcome." p.955.

42. H. C. Heins, N. W. Nance, B. J. McCarthy, C. M. Efird. "A Randomized Trial of Nurse-Midwifery Prenatal Care to Reduce Low Birth Weight." *Obstetrics and Gynecology.* 75(1990)341.

43. Oakley. "Comparisons of Maternity Care." p.823.

44. 138 Massachusetts 14 (1884).

45. 65 Florida Supp 138, 142 (DDC 1946).

46. 31 New Jersey 353, 364, 157 A2d 497, 503 (1960).

47. H. R. K. Barber. "Physicians and Lawyers: The Untapped Alliance." *Female Patient.* 20(May 1995)12.

48. Ibid.

49. Ibid.

50. Barber. "Physicians and Lawyers." p.12.

51. S. Budiansky, T. Gest, D. Fischer. "How Lawyers Abuse the Law." *Time Magazine.* 118(January 30, 1995)50.

52. Zion. "Ralph Nader. The Penthouse Interview." *Penthouse Magazine.* 26 (December 1994)83.

53. D. M. McIntosh, D. C. Murray. "The High Cost of Medical Liability." *Hudson Briefing Paper.* Number 163, April 1994.

54. Ibid.

55. Zion. "Ralph Nader. The Penthouse Interview." p.83.

56. Tillinghast, a Towers-Perrin Company. "Tort Cost Trends: An International Perspective." Tillinghast, a Towers-Perrin Company. 1992, p.1.

57. P. J. Placek, S. M. Taffel, M. Moien. "Cesarean Section Delivery Rates: United States, 1981." *American Journal of Public Health.* 73(1983)861.

58. P. J. Placek, S. M. Taffel, M. Moien. "1986 C-Sections Rise; VBAC's Inch Upward." *American Journal of Public Health.* 78(1988)562.

59. News. *Birth.* 19(September 1992)169.

60. A. R. Localio, A. G. Lawthers, J. M. Bengston, et al. "Relationship between Malpractice Claims and Cesarean Delivery." *Journal of the American Medical Association.* 269(1993)366.

61. Budiansky. "How Lawyers Abuse the Law." p.50.

62. P. W. Huber. *Galileo's Revenge.* New York: Basic Books, 1991.

63. Budiansky. "How Lawyers Abuse the Law." p.50.

64. Zion. "Ralph Nader. The Penthouse Interview." p.83.

65. R. E. Oshel, T. Croft, J. Rodak. "The National Practitioner Data Bank: The First 4 Years." *Public Health Reports.* 110(July/August 1995)383.

66. S. S. Entman, C. A. Glass, G. B. Hickson, P. B. Githens, K. W. Goldstein, F. A. Sloan. "The Relationship between Malpractice Claims History and Subsequent Obstetric Care." *Journal of the American Medical Association.* 272(1994)1588.

67. J. E. Rolph, R. L. Kravitz, K. McGuigan. "Malpractice Claims Data as a Quality Improvement Tool, II: Is Targeting Effective?" *Journal of the American Medical Association.* 266(1991)2093.

68. M. I. Taragin, F. A. Sonnenberg, M. E. Karns, R. Trout, S. Shapiro, J. L. Carson. "Does Physician Performance Explain Interspecialty Differences in Malpractice Claim Rates?" *Medical Care.* 32(1994)661.

69. S. Chapman. "Look Who's Gunning for Your Hospital Staff Privileges." *Physician's Management.* (May 1999)9.

70. *National Enquirer.* "Experts Reveal . . . Common Drug Causing Deformed Babies." *National Enquirer.* October 9, 1979, p.20.

71. Huber. "Galileo's Revenge."

72. Ibid.

73. Ibid.

74. D. A. Kessler. "The Basis of the FDA's Decision on Breast Implants." *New England Journal of Medicine.* 326(1992)1713.

75. Independent Advisory Committee on Silicone-Gel-Filled Breast Implants. "Summary of the Report on Silicone-Gel-Filled Breast Implants." *Canadian Medical Association Journal.* 147(1992)1141.

76. S. E. Gabriel, W. M. O'Fallon, L. T. Kurland, C. M. Beard, J. E. Woods, L. J. Melton. "Risk of Connective-Tissue Diseases and Other Disorders after Breast Implantation." *New England Journal of Medicine.* 330(1994)1697.

77. E. J. Giltay, H. J. Bernelot-Moens, A. H. Riley, R. G. Tan. "Silicone Breast Prostheses and Rheumatic Symptoms: A Retrospective Follow-Up Study." *Annals of Rheumatic Disease.* 53(1994)194.

78. M. H. Weisman, T. R. Vecchione, D. Albert, L. T. Moore, M. R. Mueller. "Connective-Tissue Disease Following Breast Augmentation: A Preliminary Test of the Human Adjuvant Disease Hypothesis." *Plastic and Reconstructive Surgery.* 82(1988)626.

79. A. J. Bridges, C. Conley, G. Wang, D. E. Burns, F. B. Vasey. "A Clinical and Immunologic Evaluation of Women with Silicone Breast Implants and Symptoms of Rheumatic Disease." *Annals of Internal Medicine.* 118(1993)929.

80. K. E. Wells, C. W. Cruse, J. L. Baker, et al. "The Health Status of Women Following Cosmetic Surgery." *Plastic and Reconstructive Surgery.* 93(1994)907.

81. B. L. Strom, M. M. Reidenberg, B. Freundlich, R. Schinnar. "Breast Silicone Implants and Risk of Systemic Lupus Erythematosus." *Journal of Clinical Epidemiology.* 47(1994)1211.

213

82. F. M. Wigley, R. Miller, M. C. Hochberg, V. Steen. "Augmentation Mammoplasty in Patients with Systemic Sclerosis: Data from the Baltimore Scleroderma Research Center and Pittsburgh Scleroderma Data Bank." *Arthritis and Rheumatology.* 35(1992)S-46.

83. J. A. Goldman, S. H. Lamm, W. Cooper, L. Cooper. "Breast Implants Are Not Associated with an Excess of Connective Tissue Disease." *Arthritis and Rheumatology.* 35(1992)S-65.

84. M. C. Hochberg, D. L. Perlmutter, B. White, et al. "The Association of Augmentation Mammoplasty with Systemic Sclerosis: Results from a Multi-Center Case-Control Study." *Arthritis and Rheumatology.* 37(1994)1249.

85. C. E. Dugowson, J. Daling, T. D. Koepsell, L. Voight, J. L. Nelson. "Silicone Breast Implants and Risk for Rheumatoid Arthritis." *Arthritis and Rheumatology.* 35(1992)S-66.

86. J. Sanchez-Guerrero, G. A. Colditz, E. W. Karlson, et al. "Silicone Breast Implants and the Risk of Connective-Tissue Diseases and Symptoms." *New England Journal of Medicine.* 332(1995)1666.

87. S. J. Brown. "American College of Rheumatology Defends Breast Implants." *OB/GYN News.* 30(December 15, 1995)5.

88. M. S. Webb. "Breast Deconstruction." *Contemporary Obstetrics and Gynecology.* 39(August 1994)83.

89. A. Vondrak. "Distinguished British Medical Panel Reaffirms Safety of Breast Implants." Knight-Ridder/Tribune News Service. July 13, 1998, p.713 K7884.

90. K. Dowling. "Silicone, Class-Action Nightmare." *Arizona Republic.* October 30, 1995, p.B5.

91. F. H. Boehm. "The Malpractice Scare." *MD News of Greater Phoenix.* 1(1994)8.

92. G. B. Hickson, E. W. Clayton, S. S. Entman, et al. "Obstetricians' Prior Malpractice Experience and Patients' Satisfaction with Care." *Journal of the American Medical Association.* 272(1994)1583.

93. H. B. Beckman, K. M. Markakis, A. L. Suchman, R. M. Frankel. "The Doctor-Patient Relationship and Malpractice: Lessons from Plaintiff Depositions." *Archives of Internal Medicine.* 154(June 27, 1994)1365.

94. Entman. "The Relationship between Malpractice Claims." p.1588.

95. Associated Press. "Rude Doctors Sued More, Studies Show." *New York Times.* November 25, 1994, p.B-14.

96. Budiansky. "How Lawyers Abuse the Law." p.50.

97. J. P. Phelan. "Stop the Great American Rip-off." *OB/GYN Management.* January 1995, p.6.

98. Ibid.

99. S. B. Ransom, M. P. Dombrowski, R. Shephard, M. Leonardi. "The Economic Cost of the Medical-Legal Tort System." *American Journal of Obstetrics and Gynecology.* 174(1996)1903.

100. F. A. Sloan, K. Whetten-Goldstein, G. B. Hickson. "The Influence of Obstetric No-Fault Compensation on Obstetricians' Practice Patterns." *American Journal of Obstetrics and Gynecology.* 179(1998)671.

101. F. A. Sloan, K. Whetten-Goldstein, E. M. Stout, S. S. Entman, G. B. Hickson. "No-Fault System of Compensation for Obstetric Injury: Winners and Losers." *Obstetrics and Gynecology.* 91(1998)437.

102. Phelan. "Stop the Great American Rip-off." p.6

103. Ibid.

104. Huber. *Galileo's Revenge.*

105. T. C. Rowland. "What Goes Around Comes Around." *American Journal of Obstetrics and Gynecology.* 179(August 1998)283.

106. Ibid.

107. S. S. Burstein. "Prepaid Health Care in the United States." *Illinois Medical Journal.* 160(1981)83.

108. Rowland. "What Goes Around Comes Around." p.283.

109. Ibid.

110. R. Coile. "A Short History of Capitation." *Russ Coile's Health Trends.* 8(1996)8.

111. Rowland. "What Goes Around Comes Around." p.283.

112. Ibid.

113. R. M. Cunningham. *The Healing Mission and the Business Ethic.* Chicago: Pluribus Press, 1982.

114. S. Shapiro. "An Historical Perspective on the Roots of Managed Care." *Current Opinion in Pediatrics.* 8(1996)159.

115. Rowland. "What Goes Around Comes Around." p.283.

116. D. van Amerongen. "Managed Care and Capitation." *Female Patient.* 21(February 1996)79.

117. Rowland. "What Goes Around Comes Around." p.283.

118. M. Merlin. "Congressional Research Service, Subcommittee on Health and the Environment. Appendix G. Managed Care." In *Medicaid Source Book: Background Data and Analysis.* Washington, D.C.: Government Printing Office, 1993:1009.

119. D. Chavkin, A. Treseder. "California's Prepaid Health Plan Program: Can the Patient Be Saved?" *Hastings Law Journal.* 28(1977)685.

120. D. A. Freund, R. E. Hurley. "Medicaid Managed Care: Contributions to Issues of Health Reform." *Annual Review of Public Health.* 16(1995)473.

121. D. S. Emmons, C. J. Simon. "Managed Care: Evolving Contractual Arrangements." In *Socioeconomic Characteristics of Medical Practice,* 1996. M. L. Gonzalez, editor. Chicago: American Medical Association, 1997.

122. J. Gabel. "Ten Ways HMO's Have Changed during the 1990s." *Health Affairs.* 16(1997)134.

123. G. A. Jensen, M. A. Morrisey, S. Gaffney, D. K. Liston. "The New

Dominance of Managed Care: Insurance Trends in the 1990s." *Health Affairs.* 16(1997)125.

216   124. van Amerongen. "Managed Care and Capitation." p.79.

125. M. A. Rodwin. "Conflicts in Managed Care." *New England Journal of Medicine.* 332(1995)604.

126. Ibid.

127. E. A. McGlynn. "The Effect of Managed Care on Primary Care Services for Women." *Women's Health Issues.* 8(January/February 1998)1.

128. Ibid.

129. Ibid.

130. Ibid.

131. Ibid.

132. Ibid.

133. Rodwin. "Conflicts in Managed Care." p.604.

134. S. B. Ransom, S. G. McNeeley, M. L. Kruger, G. Doot, D. B. Cotton. "The Effect of Capitated and Fee-for-Service Remuneration on Physician Decision Making in Gynecology." *Obstetrics and Gynecology.* 87(1996)707.

135. S. B. Ransom. "How Capitation Is Changing the Way We Practice." *OB/GYN Management.* August 1996, 28.

136. E. B. Smith. "FTC: Hospital Price Fixing Finds Home on the Range." *USA Today.* November 25, 1997, p.1B.

137. J. S. Gonen. "Panel Discussion." *Women's Health Issues.* 8(January/February 1998)25.

138. R. B. Gold, C. L. Richards. "Managed Care and Unintended Pregnancy." *Women's Health Issues.* 8(May/June 1998)134.

139. Associated Press. "Secret Discounts on Medical Bills Ruled Improper." *Arizona Republic.* August 31, 1995, p.A4.

140. Ibid.

141. H. R. K. Barber. "HMO's on the Ballot." *Female Patient.* 23(February 1998)9.

142. J. Castro. "Who Owns the Patient Anyway?" *Time Magazine.* July 18, 1994, p.38.

143. Ibid.

144. M. Pretzer. "Is American Medicine Overrated? These Doctors Think So." *Medical Economics.* October 5, 1998, p.35.

145. M. M. Jennings. "Clarity of Judgment during Amoral Times in a Society Addicted to Codified Law." *Otolaryngology—Head and Neck Surgery.* 117(July 1997)1.

146. J. P. Phelan. "Where Is All the Money Going?" *OB/GYN Management.* October 1998, p.8.

147. Ibid.

148. G. Espinoza. "Special Investigation: Death of an HMO." *Money.* May 1999, p.140.

149. Ibid.

150. K. Lohr. *Medicare: A Strategy for Quality Assurance.* 1. Washington, D.C.: National Academy Press, 1990.

151. J. S. Gonen. "Quality in Women's Health: Taking the Measure of Managed Care." *Insights.* July 1998, p.1.

152. OBG Management. "How the Plans Are Paying OB/GYN's." *OB/GYN Management.* January 1995, p.54.

153. G. McGrew. "A Possible Downside." *Journal of Practice Building Strategies.* Irvine, Calif.: Evergreen Group, 1995.

154. S. Parker. "ERISA May Leave Doctors as Lawsuit Targets." *OB/GYN News.* 32, Number 2(1996)53.

155. J. K. Iglehart. "Health Policy Report: Medicaid and Managed Care." *New England Journal of Medicine.* 332(1995)1727.

156. Ibid.

157. National Governors' Association. "State Medicaid Coverage of Pregnant Women and Children—Summer 1996." *MCH Update.* September 25, 1996, p.8.

158. Iglehart. "Health Policy Report." p.1727.

159. S. Schear. "A Medical Miracle?" *National Journal.* 27(1995)294.

160. A. Sharpe. "How 'Medicaid Moms' Became a Hot Market for Health Industry." *Wall Street Journal.* May 1, 1997, p.1.

161. Ibid.

162. Ibid.

163. Ibid.

164. Ibid.

165. R. H. Miller, H. S. Luft. "Managed Care Plan Performance since 1980: A Literature Analysis." *Journal of the American Medical Association.* 271(1994) 1512.

166. General Electric v. Gilbert, 45 U.S. Law Week 4031, 1976.

167. Gold. "Managed Care and Unintended Pregnancy." p.134.

168. Health Insurance Association of America. *New Group Health Insurance.* Washington, D.C.: Health Insurance Association of America, 1982.

169. McGlynn. "The Effect of Managed Care." p.1.

170. *Glamour,* Kaiser Family Foundation. Princeton Survey Research Associates. *Survey of Women about Their Knowledge, Attitudes and Practices Regarding Their Reproductive Health: A Summary of Findings.* Menlo Park, Calif.: Kaiser Family Foundation, 1997.

171. T. S. Carey, K. Weis, C. Homer. "Prepaid versus Traditional Medicaid Plans: Effects on Preventive Health Care." *Journal of Clinical Epidemiology.* 43 (1990)1213.

172. T. S. Carey, K. Weis, C. Homer. "Prepaid versus Traditional Medicaid Plans: Lack of Effect on Pregnancy Outcomes and Prenatal Care." *Health Services Research.* 26(1991)165.

218

173. T. S. Carey, K. Weis. "Diagnostic Testing and Return Visits for Acute Problems in Prepaid, Case-Managed Medicaid Plans Compared with Fee-for-Service." *Archives of Internal Medicine.* 150(1990)2369.

174. T. H. Sowell. *The Vision of the Anointed.* New York: Basic Books, 1995.

175. Gonen. "Panel Discussion." p.25.

176. T. H. Strong, W. L. Brown, W. L. Brown, C. M. Curry. "Experience with Early Post-Cesarean Hospital Dismissal." *American Journal of Obstetrics and Gynecology.* 169(1993)116.

177. Schipani. "The New Mom's Hospital Stay." p.60.

178. Strong. "Early Post-Cesarean Hospital Dismissal." p.116.

179. W. Turnbull. *Immigrant Care, Postpartum Stays, HIV Testing: Major MCH Issues in 1996.* State Reproductive Health Monitor. New York: Allan Guttmacher Institute, 1996.

180. T. H. Strong. "Maternal Postpartum Care and Hospitalization." *Clinical Consultations in Obstetrics and Gynecology.* 4(1992)277.

181. K. E. Grullon, D. A. Grimes. "The Safety of Early Postpartum Discharge: A Review and Critique." *Obstetrics and Gynecology.* 90(1997)860.

182. G. H. Olsen. Personal communication. (October 15, 1998).

183. B. Blondel. "Some Characteristics of Antenatal Care in 13 European Countries." *British Journal of Obstetrics and Gynecology.* 92(1985)565.

184. Monthly Vital Statistics Report. National Center for Health Statistics. 43, Number 5(s). Department of Health and Human Services publication number 95-1120, 4-0677. October 25, 1994.

185. "Educating Nurse-Midwives: A Strategy for Achieving Affordable, High-Quality Maternity Care." Washington, D.C.: American College of Nurse-Midwives, 1993.

186. Ibid.

187. E. S. Sekscenski, S. Sansom, C. Bazell, M. E. Salmon, F. Mullan. "State Practice Environments and the Supply of Physician Assistants, Nurse Practitioners and Certified Nurse-Midwives." *New England Journal of Medicine.* 331(1994)1266.

188. "States in Which CNM's Have Prescriptive Authority." American College of Nurse-Midwives. Publication number PR94-1/24. Washington, D.C., 1994.

189. E. A. Gravely, J. H. Littlefield. "A Cost-Effectiveness Analysis of Three Staffing Models for the Delivery of Low-Risk Prenatal Care." *American Journal of Public Health.* 82(1992)180.

190. Ibid.

191. "Educating Nurse-Midwives."

192. Ibid.

193. Ibid.

194. Schimmel. "The Yolo County Midwifery Service." p.398.

195. Blanchette. "Comparison of Obstetric Outcome." p.1864.   **219**

196. McIntosh. "The High Cost of Medical Liability."

197. Ibid.

198. Ibid.

199. E. Kinney. W. Gronfein, T. Gannon. "Indiana's Medical Malpractice Act: Results of a Three-Year Study." *Indiana Law Review*. 24, Number 3(1991) 1275.

200. D. Frum, F. Wolfe. "If You Gotta Get Sued, Get Sued in Utah." *Forbes Magazine*. January 17, 1994, p.70.

201. P. Danzon. *New Evidence on the Frequency and Severity of Medical Malpractice Claims*. Santa Monica: Rand, 1986, p.28.

202. McIntosh. "The High Cost of Medical Liability."

203. Ibid.

204. Beckman. "The Doctor-Patient Relationship." p.1365.

205. Hickson. "Factors That Prompted Families." p.1359.

206. Zion. "Ralph Nader. The Penthouse Interview." p.83.

207. Ibid.

208. E. M. Schimmel. "The Hazards of Hospitalization." *Annals of Internal Medicine*. 60(1964)100.

209. R. E. Anderson, R. B. Hill, C. R. Key. "The Sensitivity and Specificity of Clinical Diagnostics during Five Decades: Toward an Understanding of Necessary Fallibility." *Journal of the American Medical Association*. 261(1989)1610.

210. L. Goldman, R. Sayson, S. Robbins, L. H. Conn, M. Bettman, M. Weissberg. "The Value of the Autopsy in the Three Medical Eras." *New England Journal of Medicine*. 308(1983)1000.

211. H. M. Cameron, E. McGoogan. "A Prospective Study of 1152 Hospital Autopsies, I: Inaccuracies in Death Certification." *Journal of Pathology*. 133(1981) 273.

212. D. Gopher, M. Olin, Y. Donchin, et al. "The Nature and Causes of Human Errors in a Medical Intensive Care Unit." Presented at the 33rd Annual Meeting of the Human Factors Society. Denver. October 18, 1989.

213. L. L. Leape. "Error in Medicine." *Journal of the American Medical Association*. 272(1994)1851.

214. Ibid.

215. Ibid.

216. Ibid.

217. F. K. Orkin. "Patient Monitoring during Anesthesia as an Exercise in Technology Assessment." In *Monitoring in Anesthesia*. 3rd edition. L. J. Saidman, N. T. Smith, editors. London: Butterworth Publishers, 1993.

218. F. A. Sloan, P. M. Mergenhagen, B. Burfield, R. R. Boubjerg, M. Hassan.

"Medical Malpractice Experience of Physicians: Predictable or Haphazard?" *Journal of the American Medical Association*. 262(1989)3291.

220   219. T. Sagin. "Are Primary Care Physicians Riding the Crest or Entering the Trough?" *Healthcare Leadership Review*. September 1998, p.4.

220. J. J. Fangman, P. M. Mark, L. Pratt, et al. "Prematurity Prevention Programs: An Analysis of Successes and Failures." *American Journal of Obstetrics and Gynecology*. 170(1994)744.

221. R. Brannon, S. Orrick. "Women and Managed Care: The Employer's Perspective." *Women's Health Issues*. 8(January/February 1998)15.

222. Gonen. "Quality in Women's Health." p. 1.

223. L. B. McCullough, F. A. Chervenak. "Ethical Challenges in the Managed Practice of Obstetrics and Gynecology." *Obstetrics and Gynecology*. 93(1999)304.

224. K. G. Burke, S. J. Schwartz. "Profit over Patients?" *C and D Quarterly*. 1(Spring/Summer 1998)1.

225. W. J. Guglielmo. "How Monica Maria Stalled HMO Reform." *Medical Economics*. December 28, 1998, p.23.

226. Ibid.

227. Ibid.

228. Pretzer. "Is American Medicine Overrated?" p.35.

229. K. Cheney. "What You Can Learn from an MD Mutiny in a Managed-Care Plan." *Money Magazine*. December 1995, p.21.

230. Rodwin. "Conflicts in Managed Care." p.604.

231. Cheney. "What You Can Learn from an MD Mutiny." p.21.

232. Ibid.

233. Ibid.

234. Ibid.

NOTES TO CHAPTER 5

1. D. Popenoe. "Family Caps." *Society*. 33(July/August 1996)25.

2. S. M. Dornbusch, M. R. Herman, I. C. Lin. "Single Parenthood." *Society*. 33(July/August 1996)30.

3. C. K. Mrela. *Arizona Health Status and Vital Statistics, 1995*. Phoenix: Arizona Department of Health Services, 1996.

4. Popenoe. "Family Caps." p.25.

5. J. C. Gersten, C. K. Mrela. *Closing the Decade: Arizona Health Status and Vital Statistics, 1980–1989*. Phoenix: Arizona Department of Health Services, 1990.

6. S. B. Amini, L. J. Dierker, P. M. Catalano, G. G. Ashmead, L. I. Mann. "Trends in an Obstetric Patient Population: An Eighteen-Year Study." *American Journal of Obstetrics and Gynecology*. 171(1994)1014.

7. H. G. Schneiderman. "Antisocial Personalities, Antidemocratic Solutions." *Society.* 33(November/December 1996)53.

8. Ibid.

9. Ibid.

10. Ibid.

11. Ibid.

12. Ibid.

13. Ibid.

14. Ibid.

15. A. B. Berenson, N. J. Stiglich, G. S. Wilkinson, G. D. Anderson. "Drug Abuse and Other Risk Factors for Physical Abuse in Pregnancy among White Non-Hispanic, Black and Hispanic Women." *American Journal of Obstetrics and Gynecology.* 164(1991)1491.

16. L. F. Bullock, J. McFarlane. "The Birthweight/Battering Connection." *American Journal of Nursing.* 89(1989)1153.

17. J. Golding, J. Henriques, P. Thomas. "Unmarried at Delivery, II, Perinatal Morbidity and Mortality." *Early Human Development.* 14(1986)217.

18. L. J. McIntosh, N. E. Roumayah, S. F. Bottoms. "Perinatal Outcome of Broken Marriage in the Inner-City." *Obstetrics and Gynecology.* 85(1995)233.

19. R. J. Herrnstein, C. Murray. *The Bell Curve.* New York: Free Press, 1994, p.181.

20. Ibid. p.215.

21. E. H. Quint. "Adolescent Pregnancy: An Update." *Female Patient.* 21(1996)15.

22. S. J. Ventura, K. D. Peters, J. A. Martin, J. D. Maurer. *Births and Deaths: United States, 1996.* Monthly Vital Statistics Report. Supplement. Volume 46, Number 1. Hyattsville, Md.: National Center for Health Statistics, 1997.

23. Dornbusch. "Single Parenthood." p.30.

24. J. Trussell. "Teenage Pregnancy in the United States." *Family Planning Perspectives.* 20(1988)262.

25. Dornbusch. "Single Parenthood." p.30.

26. A. Friede, W. Baldwin, P. H. Rhoades, et al. "Young Maternal Age and Infant Mortality: The Role of Low Birth Weight." *Public Health Report.* 102(1987) 192.

27. H. L. Brown, Y. D. Fan, W. J. Gonsoulin. "Obstetric Complications in Young Teenagers." *Southern Medical Journal.* 84(1991)46.

28. Quint. "Adolescent Pregnancy." p.15.

29. M. L. Blankson, S. P. Cliver, R. L. Goldenberg, C. A. Hickey, J. Jin, M. B. Dubard. "Health Behavior and Outcomes in Sequential Pregnancies of Black and White Adolescents." *Journal of the American Medical Association.* 269(1993) 1401.

221

30. S. J. Ventura, J. A. Martin, S. C Curtin, T. J. Mathews. *Report of Final Natality Statistics, 1995*. Monthly Vital Statistics Report. Supplement. Volume 45, Number 11. Hyattsville, Md.: National Center for Health Statistics, 1997.

31. A. M. Fraser, J. E. Brockert, R. H. Ward. "Association of Young Maternal Age with Adverse Reproductive Outcomes." *New England Journal of Medicine.* 332(1995)1113.

32. C. Sowers. "Arizona High in Teen-Age Sex." *Arizona Republic.* May 6, 1995, p.A1.

33. *New York Times.* "Teenage Birth Rates on Decline." *Arizona Republic.* January 5, 1997, p.A11.

34. L. Meckler (Associated Press). "Teen Birth, Abortion Rates Decrease across Country." *Arizona Republic.* June 27, 1998, p.A30.

35. Alan Guttmacher Institute. *Sex and America's Teenagers.* New York: Alan Guttmacher Institute, 1994.

36. Meckler. "Teen Birth." p.A30.

37. S. Stolberg. "Small Town Targets Teen Sex." *Arizona Republic.* December 1, 1996, p.A15.

38. K. Painter. "Fewer Teens Having Sex; More Use Birth Control." USA Today. May 2, 1997, p.D1. A common game which is played with statistics deserves mention here because it applies to our discussion. While it is true that America's teenage pregnancy rate is finally on the decline, the actual magnitude of the decline is open to political interpretation. To illustrate, our teenage pregnancy rate fell from a high of 61 percent in 1991 to 56 percent in 1995. Among those wishing to downplay the improvement, a 5-percent absolute drop in the rate could be cited. On the other hand, the five-point drop could be presented by those wishing to optimize the effect as a percentage of the 61-percent rate reported in 1991 (e.g., $5 \div 61 = 8.2$ percent), thereby giving the impression that the relative drop in our teen pregnancy rate is nearly double that of the absolute drop.

39. E. Goodman. "It's Time to Revive the Word 'Jailbait.'" *Arizona Republic.* February 22, 1995, p.B5.

40. L. Valdez. "The Legislative Assault on Little Girls Won't Curb Teen Pregnancy." *Arizona Republic.* November 3, 1995, p.B5.

41. Ibid.

42. M. Charen. "Revealing Picture of Teen Sex Emerges." *Fresno Bee.* August 10, 1995, p.B7.

43. M. D. Benson, E. J. Torpy. "Sexual Behavior in Junior High School Students." *Obstetrics and Gynecology.* 85(1995)279.

44. Charen. "Revealing Picture." p.B7.

45. D. Boyer, D. Fine. "Sexual Abuse as a Factor in Adolescent Pregnancy and Child Maltreatment." *Family Planning Perspectives.* 24(1992)11.

46. M. Males. "Adult Liaison in the 'Epidemic' of 'Teenage' Birth, Pregnancy and Venereal Disease." *Journal of Sexual Research.* 29(1992)525.

47. J. B. Hardy, A. K. Duggan. "Teenage Fathers and the Fathers of Infants of Urban Teenage Mothers." *American Journal of Public Health.* 78(1988) 919.

48. D. J. Landry, J. D. Forrest. "How Old Are U.S. Fathers?" *Family Planning Perspectives.* 27(1995)159.

49. Allan Guttmacher Institute. *Teenage Pregnancy and Births in California: Trends and Characteristics.* New York: Alan Guttmacher Institute, 1994.

50. F. Sonenstein. "Risking Paternity: Sex and Contraception among Adolescent Males." In *Adolescent Fatherhood.* A. Elsters, M. Lamb, editors. Hillsdale, N.J.: Lawrence Erlbaum Associates, 1986.

51. G. Adams, K. Pittman, R. O'Brien. "Adolescent and Young Fathers: Problems and Solutions." In *The Politics of Pregnancy: Adolescent Sexuality and Public Policy.* A. Lawson, D. L. Rhode, editors. Ann Arbor, Mich.: Edward Brothers, Inc., 1993.

52. Males. "Adult Liaison in the 'Epidemic' of 'Teenage' Birth." p.525.

53. Landry. "How Old Are U.S. Fathers?" p.159.

54. M. E. Lamb, A. B. Elsters, J. Travare. "Behavioral Profiles of Adolescent Mothers and Partners with Varying Intracouple Age Differences." *Journal of Adolescent Research.* 1(1986)399.

55. Ibid.

56. Ibid.

57. D. Taylor, G. Chavez, A. Chabra, J. Boggess. "Risk Factors for Adult Paternity in Births to Adolescents." *Obstetrics and Gynecology.* 89(1997)199.

58. A. B. Elsters, M. E. Lamb, N. Kimmerly. "Perceptions of Parenthood among Adolescent Fathers." *Pediatrics.* 83(1989)452.

59. I. I. Nakashima, B. W. Camp. "Fathers of Infants Born to Adolescent Mothers." *American Journal of Disease in Children.* 138(1984)452.

60. F. Ahmed, J. A. McRae, N. Ahmed. "Factors Associated with Not Receiving Adequate Prenatal Care in an Urban Black Population: Program Planning Implications." *Social Work in Health Care.* 14(1990)107.

61. G. R. Alexander, G. Baruffi, J. M. Mor, E. C. Kieffer, T. C. Hulsey. "Multiethnic Variations in the Pregnancy Outcomes of Military Dependents." *American Journal of Public Health.* 83(1993)1721.

62. R. E. Zambrana, C. Dunkel-Schetter, S. Scrimshaw. "Factors Which Influence Use of Prenatal Care in Low-Income Racial-Ethnic Women in Los Angeles County." *Journal of Community Health.* 16(October 1991)283.

63. R. Palkovitz. "Fathers' Motives for Birth Attendance." *Maternal and Child Nursing Journal.* 16(1987)123.

64. R. J. Revak-Lutz, K. R. Kellner. "Paternal Involvement after Perinatal Death." *Journal of Perinatology.* 14(1994)442.

65. Zambrana. "Factors Which Influence Use of Prenatal Care." p.283.

66. F. D. Martinez, A. L. Wright, L. M. Taussig, Group Health Medical

NOTES TO CHAPTER 5

Associates. "The Effect of Paternal Smoking on the Birthweight of Newborns Whose Mothers Did Not Smoke." *American Journal of Public Health.* 84(1994) 1489.

67. B. Bergman, G. Larsson, B. Brismar, M. Klang. "Aetiological and Precipitating Factors in Wife Battering." *Acta Psychiatry of Scandinavia.* 77(1988)338.

68. Gersten. *Closing the Decade.* p.33.

69. M. L. Nordstrom, S. Cnattingius, B. Haglund. "Social Differences in Swedish Infant Mortality by Cause of Death, 1983 to 1986." *American Journal of Public Health.* 83(1993)26.

70. J. E. Miller. "Birth Intervals and Perinatal Health: An Investigation of Three Hypotheses." *Family Planning Perspectives.* 23(1991)62.

71. Nordstrom. "Social Differences." p.26.

72. U. Hogberg, S. Wall, D. E. Wiklun. "Perinatal Mortality in a Swedish County, 1980–1984. Mortality Pattern and Its Amendability." *Acta Obstetrics and Gynecology of Scandinavia.* 69(1990)567.

73. B. Nold, R. A. Stallones, W. E. Reynolds. "The Social Class Gradient of Perinatal Mortality in Dependents of Military Personnel." *American Journal of Epidemiology.* 83(1966)481.

74. J. B. Gould, S. LeRoy. "Socioeconomic Status and Low Birth Weight: A Racial Comparison." *Pediatrics.* 82(1988)896.

75. E. S. Fisher, J. P. LoGerfo, J. R. Daling. "Prenatal Care and Pregnancy Outcomes during the Recession: The Washington State Experience." *American Journal of Public Health.* 75(1985)866.

76. D. Baird. "The Epidemiology of Prematurity." *Journal of Pediatrics.* 64(1964)909.

77. T. F. Porter, A. M. Fraser, C. Y. Hunter, R. H. Ward, M. W. Varner. "The Risk of Preterm Birth across Generations." *Obstetrics and Gynecology.* 90(1997)63.

78. News of Note. "U.S. STD Rate Highest in Developed World." *Female Patient.* 22(1997)12.

79. J. M. Piper, E. R. Newton, R. N. Shain, S. T. Perdue, J. H. Dimmitt. "Does Pregnancy Offer an Added Incentive for Risk Reduction to Avoid Sexually Transmitted Diseases?" *American Journal of Obstetrics and Gynecology.* 176, Number 1, Part 2(176)538.

80. P. J. Meis, J. M. Ernest, M. L. Moore. "Causes of Low Birth Weight Births in Public and Private Patients." *American Journal of Obstetrics and Gynecology.* 156(1987)1165.

81. Amini. "Trends in an Obstetric Patient Population." p.1014.

82. *Income Mobility and Economic Opportunity.* Report prepared for Representative Richard K. Armey, Ranking Republican. Joint Economic Committee. June 1992, p.5.

83. G. J. Duncan, et al. *Years of Poverty, Years of Plenty: The Changing Economic Fortunes of American Workers and Families.* Ann Arbor: University of Michigan

Press, 1984.

84. N. Gilbert. "Welfare Reform Priorities." *Society.* 33(July/August 1996)43.

85. The Panel Study of Income Dynamics (PSID) is an ongoing, longitudinal **225** study of American households which was initiated in 1968 by the Survey Research Center at the University of Michigan.

86. W. E. Williams. "The Welfare Debate." *Society.* 33(July/August 1996)13.

87. Gilbert. "Welfare Reform Priorities." p.43.

88. S. E. Mayer. *What Money Can't Buy: Family Income and Children's Life Chances.* Cambridge: Harvard University Press, 1997.

89. L. M. Mead. "Welfare Reform at Work." *Society.* 33(July/August 1996)37.

90. Gilbert. "Welfare Reform Priorities." p.43.

91. Ibid.

92. Ibid.

93. B. M. Roth. "Crime and Child-Rearing." *Society.* 33(November/December 1996)40.

94. Ibid.

95. Mead. "Welfare Reform at Work." p.37.

96. K. Bland. "Second Look at Aiding Abused Children." *Arizona Republic.* February 17, 1997, p.A1.

97. United States Department of Health and Human Services. *Healthy People 2000: National Health Promotion and Disease Prevention Objectives.* DHHS publication number PHS 91-50212. Washington, D.C.: United States Department of Health and Human Services, Public Health Service, 1991.

98. J. Heller, H. R. Anderson, J. M. Bland, et al. "Alcohol in Pregnancy: Patterns and Association with Socio-Economic, Psychological and Behavioral Factors." *British Journal of Addiction.* 83(1983)541.

99. J. S. Knisely, E. R. Spear, D. J. Green, et al. "Substance Abuse Patterns in Pregnant Women." *NIDA Research Monogram.* 105(1991)280.

100. F. F. Broekhuizen, J. Utrie, C. Van Mullem. "Drug Use or Inadequate Prenatal Care? Adverse Pregnancy Outcome in an Urban Setting." *American Journal of Obstetrics and Gynecology.* 166(1992)1747.

101. B. M. Aved, M. M. Irwin, L. S. Cummings, N. Findiesen. "Barriers to Prenatal Care for Low-Income Women." *Western Journal of Medicine.* 158(1993) 493.

102. T. Joyce, A. D. Racine. "An Update on New York City's Dramatic Increase in Low Birthweight." *American Journal of Public Health.* 83(1993)109.

103. S. H. Ebrahim, E. T. Luman, R. L. Floyd, C. C. Murphy, E. M. Bennett, C. A. Boyle. "Alcohol Consumption by Pregnant Women in the United States during 1988–1995." *Obstetrics and Gynecology.* 92(1998)187.

104. C. M. Wiemann, A. B. Berenson, V. V. San Miguel. "Tobacco, Alcohol and Illicit Drug Use among Pregnant Women: Age and Racial/Ethnic Differences." *Journal of Reproductive Medicine.* 39(1994)769.

105. Berenson. "Drug Abuse and Other Risk Factors." p.1491.

106. J. Ager, S. Martier, J. Sloan, J. Hankin, I. Firestone, R. Sokol. "Recent Trends in Maternal Drinking for an Inner-City Clinic Population." *American Journal of Obstetrics and Gynecology*. 164, Number 1, Part 2(1991)410.

107. V. R. Lupo, P. S. Kapernick. "Effect of Substance Abuse Reporting Laws on Cocaine Use in Subsequent Pregnancies." *American Journal of Obstetrics and Gynecology*. 166, Number 1, Part 2(1992)305.

108. M. D. Peoples-Sheps, W. D. Kalsbeek, E. Siegel, C. Dewees, M. Rogers, R. Schwartz. "Prenatal Records: A National Survey of Content." *American Journal of Obstetrics and Gynecology*. 164(1991)514.

109. Broekhuizen. "Drug Use or Inadequate Prenatal Care?" p.1747.

110. Ibid.

111. D. E. McLean, K. Hatfield-Timajchy, P. A. Wingo, R. L. Floyd. "Psychosocial Measurement: Implications for the Study of Preterm Delivery in Black Women." In "Racial Differences in Preterm Delivery, Developing a New Research Paradigm." *American Journal of Preventive Medicine*. Supplement. Volume 9, Number 6(November/December 1993)39.

112. J. S. Norbeck, N. J. Anderson. "Psychosocial Predictors of Pregnancy Outcomes in Low-Income Black, Hispanic and White Women." *Nursing Research*. 38(1989)204.

113. McLean. "Psychosocial Measurement." p.39.

114. Ibid.

115. J. E. Dimsdale, J. Moss. "Plasma Catecholamines in Stress and Exercise." *Journal of the American Medical Association*. 243(1980)340.

116. S. Cohen, G. M. Williamson. "Stress and Infectious Disease in Humans." Psychology Bulletin. 109(1991)205.

117. C. N. Ramsey, T. D. Abell, L. C. Baker. "The Relationship between Family Functioning, Life Events, Family Structure and the Outcome of Pregnancy." *Journal of Family Practice*. 22(1986)521.

118. C. J. Hobel, C. Dunkel-Schetter, S. Roesch. "Maternal Stress as a Signal to the Fetus." *Prenatal and Neonatal Medicine*. 3(1998)116.

119. C. Dunkel-Schetter. "Maternal Stress and Preterm Delivery." *Prenatal and Neonatal Medicine*. 3(1998)39.

120. A. J. Beck, D. K. Gilliard. "Prisoners in 1994." *Bureau of Justice Statistics Bulletin*. NCJ-151654. August 1995.

121. T. L. Snell, D. C. Morton. "Women in Prison: Survey of State Prison Inmates, 1991." *Bureau of Justice Statistics Special Report*. March 1994.

122. P. J. Elton. "Mothers and Babies in Prison." *Lancet*. 1(1987)501.

123. D. Mellor. *Parliamentary Written Answer*. Number 71, 1986.

124. P. J. Elton. "Outcome of Pregnancy amongst Prisoners." *Journal of Obstetrics and Gynecology*. 5(1985)241.

226

125. J. V. Terk, M. G. Martens, M. A. Williamson. "Pregnancy Outcomes of Incarcerated Women." *Journal of Maternal-Fetal Medicine.* 2(1993)246.

126. D. R. Mishell, T. H. Kirschbeum, C. P. Morrow. *The Year Book of Obstetrics and Gynecology.* St. Louis: Mosby, 1993, p.49. **227**

127. L. Cordero, S. Hines, K. A. Shibley, M. B. Landon. "Perinatal Outcome for Women in Prison." *Journal of Perinatology.* 12(1992)205.

128. C. C. Egley, D. E. Miller, J. L. Granados, C. Ingram-Fogel. "Outcome of Pregnancy during Imprisonment." *Journal of Reproductive Medicine.* 37(1992) 131.

129. S. L. Martin, H. Kim, L. L. Kupper, R. E. Meyer, M. Hays. "Is Incarceration during Pregnancy Associated with Infant Birthweight?" *American Journal of Public Health.* 87(1997)1526.

130. J. Pasternak. "Wisconsin OK's Civil Detention for Fetal Abuse." *Los Angeles Times.* May 2, 1998, p.A1.

131. Ibid.

132. E. D. Peterson, S. M. Wright, J. Daley, G. E. Thibault. "Racial Variation in Cardiac Procedure Use and Survival Following Acute Myocardial Infarction in the Department of Veteran Affairs. *Journal of the American Medical Association.* 271(1994)1175.

133. J. Whittle, J. Conigliaro, C. B. Good, R. P. Lofgren. "Racial Differences in the Use of Invasive Cardiovascular Procedures in the Department of Veterans Affairs Medical System." *New England Journal of Medicine.* 329(1993)621.

134. H. J. Geiger. "Race and Health Care—An American Dilemma." *New England Journal of Medicine.* 335(1996)815.

135. R. S. Gaston, I. Ayres, L. G. Dooley, A. G. Diethelm. "Racial Equality in Renal Transplantation." *Journal of the American Medical Association.* 270(1993) 1352.

136. A. M. McBean, M. Gornick. "Differences by Race in the Rates of Procedures Performed in Hospitals for Medicare Beneficiaries." *Health Care Financial Review.* 15, Number 4(1994)77.

137. J. J. Escarce, K. R. Epstein, D. C. Colby, J. S. Schwartz. "Racial Differences in the Elderly's Use of Medical Procedures and Diagnostic Tests." *American Journal of Public Health.* 83(1993)948.

138. M. E. Gornick, P. W. Eggers, T. W. Reilly, et al. "Effects of Race and Income on Mortality and Use of Services among Medicare Beneficiaries." *New England Journal of Medicine.* 335(1996)791.

139. Physician Payment Review Commission. *Monitoring Access of Medicare Beneficiaries.* Report 92-5. Washington, D.C.: Physician Payment Review Commission, 1992.

140. S. J. Ventura, J. A. Martin, S. M. Taffel, T. J. Mathews, S. C. Clarke. *Advance Report of Final Natality Statistics,* 1992. Monthly Vital Statistics Report.

Supplement. Volume 43, Number 5. Hyattsville, Md.: National Center for Health Statistics, 1994.

228   141. Gersten. *Closing the Decade.*

142. Mrela. *Arizona Health Status.*

143. Gersten. *Closing the Decade.*

144. Mrela. *Arizona Health Status.*

145. Ibid.

146. Gersten. *Closing the Decade.*

147. M. E. Wegman. "Annual Summary of Vital Statistics—1992." *Pediatrics.* 92(1993)743.

148. B. Guyer, J. A. Martin, M. F. MacDorman, R. N. Anderson, D. M. Strobino. "Annual Summary of Vital Statistics—1996." *Pediatrics.* 100(1997) 905.

149. B. Guyer, M. F. MacDorman, J. A. Martin, K. D. Peters, D. M. Strobino. "Annual Summary of Vital Statistics—1997." *Pediatrics.* 102(1998)1333.

150. J. A. Horton. *State Profiles on Women's Health.* Washington, D.C.: Jacobs Institute of Women's Health, 1998, p.4.

151. Mrela. *Arizona Health Status.*

152. Amini. "Trends in an Obstetric Patient Population." p.1014.

153. S. K. Virji, E. Cottington. "Risk Factors Associated with Preterm Deliveries among Racial Groups in a National Sample of Married Mothers." *American Journal of Perinatology.* 8(1991)347.

154. S. M. Taffel. "Trends in Low Birth Weight: United States, 1975–87." National Center for Health Statistics. *Vital Health Statistics.* 21(48)1989.

155. Guyer. "Annual Summary of Vital Statistics—1997." p.1333.

156. K. C. Schoendorf, C. J. R. Hogue, J. C. Kleinman, D. Rowley. "Mortality among Infants of Black as Compared with White College-Educated Parents." *New England Journal of Medicine.* 326(1992)1522.

157. P. Petitti, C. Coleman, D. Binsacca, et al. "Early Prenatal Care in Urban Black and White Women." *Birth.* 17(1990)1.

158. R. Ferguson, S. A. Myers. "The Effect of Race on the Relationship between Fetal Death and Altered Fetal Growth." *American Journal of Obstetrics and Gynecology.* 163(1990)1222.

159. R. L. Copper, R. L. Goldenberg, M. B. DuBard, R. O. Davis, The Collaborative Group on Preterm Birth Prevention. "Risk Factors for Fetal Death in White, Black and Hispanic Women." *Obstetrics and Gynecology.* 84(1994)490.

160. M. M. Adams, J. A. Read, J. S. Rawlings, F. B. Harlass, A. P. Sarno, P. H. Rhodes. "Preterm Delivery among Black and White Enlisted Women in the United States Army." *Obstetrics and Gynecology.* 81(1993)65.

161. M. M. Adams, F. B. Harlass, A. P. Sarno, J. A. Read, J. S. Rawlings. "Antenatal Hospitalization among Enlisted Servicewomen, 1987—1990." *Obstetrics and Gynecology.* 84(1994)35.

162. J. S. Rawlings, M. R. Weir. "Race and Rank-Specific Infant Mortality in a U.S. Military Population." *American Journal of Diseases of Children*. 146(1992) 313.

163. A. C. Miller. "Infant Mortality in the United States." *Scientific American*. 253(1985)31.

164. G. K. Singh, S. M. Yu. "Infant Mortality in the United States: Trends, Differentials and Projections, 1950 through 2010." *American Journal of Public Health*. 85(1995)957.

165. Guyer. "Annual Summary of Vital Statistics—1997." p.1333.

166. J. E. Becerra, C. J. Hogue, H. K. Atrash, N. Perez. "Infant Mortality among Hispanics—A Portrait of Heterogeneity." *Journal of the American Medical Association*. 265(1991)217.

167. R. Scribner, J. H. Dwyer. "Acculturation and Low Birthweight among Latinos in the Hispanic HANES." *American Journal of Public Health*. 79(1989) 1263.

168. F. A. Hayek. *Law, Legislation and Liberty*. Chicago: University of Chicago Press, 1973.

169. S. A. James. "Racial and Ethnic Differences in Infant Mortality and Low Birth Weight: A Psychosocial Critique." *Annals of Epidemiology*. 3(1993)130.

170. A. E. Camilli, L. F. McElroy, K. L. Reed. "Smoking and Pregnancy: A Comparison of Mexican-American and Non-Hispanic White Women." *Obstetrics and Gynecology*. 84(1994)1033.

171. G. Marin, F. Sabogal, B. Marin, R. Otero-Sabogal, E. J. Perez-Stable. "Development of a Short Acculturation Scale for Hispanics." *Hispanic Journal of Behavioral Science*. 9(1987)183.

172. Wiemann. "Tobacco, Alcohol and Illicit Drug Use." p.769.

173. R. D. Lamm. "Healthcare Heresies." *Healthcare Forum Journal*. (September/October 1994)45.

174. J. C. Kleinman, L. A. Fingerhut, K. Prager. "Differences in Infant Mortality by Race, Nativity Status and Other Maternal Characteristics." *American Journal of Diseases of Children*. 145(1991)194.

175. S. Taffel. *Factors Associated with Low Birth Weight*. Series 21, Number 37. Publication number (PHS) 80:1915. Hyattsville, Md.: National Center for Health Statistics, 1980.

176. H. Cabral, L. E. Fried, S. Levenson, H. Amaro, B. Zuckerman. "Foreign-Born and U.S.-Born Black Women: Differences in Health Behaviors and Birth Outcomes." *American Journal of Public Health*. 80(1990)70.

177. F. Barros. "An International Perspective: Brazil and Cuba." Presented at Preterm Delivery among Black Women: The Symposium on Psychosocial Factors. Atlanta. December 5, 1991.

178. F. Rasmussen, C. E. M. Oldenburg, A. Ericson, J. Gunnarskog. "Preterm

Birth and Low Birthweight among Children of Swedish and Immigrant Women between 1978 and 1990." *Paediatric and Perinatal Epidemiology.* 9(1995)441.

179. H. Wasse, V. L. Holt, J. R. Daling. "Pregnancy Risk Factors and Birth Outcomes in Washington State: A Comparison of Ethiopian-Born and U.S.-Born Women." *American Journal of Public Health.* 9(1994)1505.

180. Camilli. "Smoking and Pregnancy." p.1033.

181. P. A. Buescher, C. Smith, J. L. Holliday, R. H. Levine. "Source of Prenatal Care and Infant Birth Weight: The Case of a North Carolina County." *American Journal of Obstetrics and Gynecology.* 156(1987)204.

182. James. "Racial and Ethnic Differences." p.130.

183. M. D. Kogan, M. Kotelchuck, G. R. Alexander, W. E. Johnson. "Racial Disparities in Reported Prenatal Care Advice from Health Care Providers." *American Journal of Public Health.* 84(1994)82.

184. Zambrana. "Factors Which Influence Use of Prenatal Care." p.283.

185. K. M. Brett, K. C. Schoendorf, J. L. Keily. "Differences between Black and White Women in the Use of Prenatal Care Technologies." *American Journal of Obstetrics and Gynecology.* 170(1994)41.

186. M. N. Bustan, A. L. Coker. "Maternal Attitude toward Pregnancy and the Risk of Neonatal Death." *American Journal of Public Health.* 84(1994)411.

187. A. Myhrman. "The Northern Finland Cohort, 1966–82: A Follow-Up Study of Children Unwanted at Birth." In H. P. David, Z. Dytrych, Z. Matejcek, V. Schuller, editors. *Born Unwanted.* New York: Springer, 1988, p.103.

188. M. Schlesinger, K. Dronebusch. "The Failure of Prenatal Care Policy for the Poor." *Health Affairs.* 9(Winter 1990)91.

189. M. L. Poland, J. Ager, J. Olson. "Barriers to Receiving Adequate Prenatal Care." *American Journal of Obstetrics and Gynecology.* 157(1987)297.

190. R. H. Weller, I. W. Eberstein, M. Bailey. "Pregnancy Wantedness and Maternal Behavior during Pregnancy." *Demography.* 24(August 1987)407.

191. K. Joyce, G. Diffenbacher, J. Greene, Y. Sorokin. "Internal and External Barriers to Obtaining Prenatal Care." *Social Work in Health Care.* 9(1983)89.

192. D. A. Nagey. "The Content of Prenatal Care." *Obstetrics and Gynecology.* 74(1989)516.

193. The Coronary Drug Project Research Group. "Influence of Adherence to Treatment." *New England Journal of Medicine.* 303(1980)1038.

194. G. Lindmark, S. Cnattingius. "The Scientific Basis of Antenatal Care: Report from a State-of-the-Art Conference." *Acta Obstetrics and Gynecology of Scandinavia.* 70(1991)105.

195. Weller. "Pregnancy Wantedness." p.407.

196. J. Yerushalmy. "The Relationship of Parents' Cigarette Smoking to Outcome of Pregnancy—Implication as to the Problem of Inferring Causation from Observed Associations." *American Journal of Epidemiology.* 93(1971)443.

197. S. Kullander, B. Kallen. "A Prospective Study of Smoking and Pregnancy." *Acta Obstetrica et Gynecologica Scandinavica.* 50(1971)83.

198. Morbidity and Mortality Weekly Report. "Unintended Childbearing: **231** Pregnancy Risk Assessment Monitoring System—Oklahoma." *Morbidity and Mortality Weekly Report.* 41(1992)933.

199. S. F. Meikle, M. Orleans, M. Leff, R. Shain, R. S. Gibbs. "Women's Reasons for Not Seeking Prenatal Care: Racial and Ethnic Factors." *Birth.* 22 (1995)81.

200. R. L. Cohen. "Maladaptation to Pregnancy." *Seminars in Perinatology.* 3(1979)15.

201. Petitti. "Early Prenatal Care." p.1.

202. P. Finnegan, E. McKinstry, G. E. Robinson. "Denial of Pregnancy and Childbirth." *Canadian Journal of Psychiatry.* 27(1982)672.

203. P. Soloff, S. Jewell, L. Roth. "Civil Commitment and the Rights of the Unborn." *American Journal of Psychiatry.* 136(1979)114.

204. M. Brozosky. H. Falit. "Neonaticide: Clinical and Psychosomatic Considerations." *Journal of the American Academy of Child and Adolescent Psychiatry.* 27 (1971)673.

205. A. M. Spielvogel, H. C. Hohener. "Denial of Pregnancy: A Review and Case Reports." *Birth.* 22(1995)220.

206. E. R. Pamuk, W. D. Mosher. *Health Aspects of Pregnancy and Childbirth, United States, 1982.* DHHS publication number 89-1992. Hyattsville, Md.: Department of Health and Human Services, 1982.

207. H. A. Hein. "Do We Have the Infant Mortality Rate We Desire?" *Journal of the American Medical Association.* 266(1991)114.

208. B. Ferguson. "Health Care Access and Birth Outcome." *Journal of the American Medical Association.* 269(1993)2506.

209. L. Rajan, A. Oakley. "Low Birthweight Babies: The Mother's Point of View." *Midwifery.* 6(1990)73.

210. M. P. Laken, J. Ager. "Using Incentives to Increase Participation in Prenatal Care." *Obstetrics and Gynecology.* 85(1995)326.

211. J. M. Lang, E. Lieberman, K. J. Ryan, R. R. Monson. "Interpregnancy Interval and Risk of Preterm Labor." *American Journal of Epidemiology.* 132(1990) 304.

212. J. S. Rawlings, V. B. Rawlings, J. A. Read. "Prevalence of Low Birth Weight and Preterm Delivery in Relation to the Interval between Pregnancies among White and Black Women." *New England Journal of Medicine.* 332 (1995)69.

213. O. Basso, J. Olsen, L. B. Knudsen, K. Christensen. "Low Birth Weight and Preterm Birth after Short Interpregnancy Intervals." *American Journal of Obstetrics and Gynecology.* 178(1998)259.

214. P. C. Leppert. "Factors Contributing to Japan's Low Infant Mortality

Rate." *American Journal of Obstetrics and Gynecology.* 168, Number 1, Part 2 (1993)366.

232   215. Ibid.

216. M. I. Evans, E. Gleicher, M. P. Johnson, R. J. Sokol. "The Fiscal Impact of the Medicaid Abortion Funding Ban in Michigan." *American Journal of Obstetrics and Gynecology.* 166, Number 1, Part 2(1992)397.

217. M. Grossman, S. Jacobowitz. "Variations in Infant Mortality Rates among Counties of the United States." *Demography.* 18(1981)695.

218. A. Torres, P. Donovan, N. Dittes, J. D. Forrest. "Public Benefits and Costs of Government Funding for Abortion." *Family Planning Perspectives.* 18(1986) 111.

219. K. J. Meier, D. R. McFarlane. "State Family Planning and Abortion Expenditures: Their Effect on Public Health." *American Journal of Public Health.* 84(1994)9.

220. T. J. Joyce, M. Grossman. "The Dynamic Relationship between Low Birthweight and Induced Abortion in New York City: An Aggregate Time-Series Analysis." *Journal of Home Economics.* 9(1990)273.

221. D. J. Jamieson, P. A. Buescher. "The Effect of Family Planing Participation on Prenatal Care Use and Low Birthweight." *Family Planning Perspectives.* 24 (1992)214.

222. D. Rosenak, H. Yaffe, E. Voss, Y. Shiklosh, Y. Levy, E. Hornstein. "Outcome of Pregnancies Destined for Adoption." *American Journal of Obstetrics and Gynecology.* 164, Number 1, Part 2(1991)286.

223. P. H. Wise. "Confronting Racial Disparities in Infant Mortality: Reconciling Science and Politics." In "Racial Differences in Preterm Delivery: Developing a New Research Paradigm." *American Journal of Preventive Medicine.* Supplement. Volume 9, Number 6 (November/December 1993)7.

224. Guyer. "Annual Summary—1996." p.905.

225. P. H. Shiono, V. A. Rauh, M. Park, et al. "Ethnic Differences in Birthweight: The Role of Lifestyle and Other Factors." *American Journal of Public Health.* 87(1997)787.

226. J. V. Van Der Merwe. "Physician-Patient Communication Using Ancestral Spirits to Achieve Holistic Healing." *American Journal of Obstetrics and Gynecology.* 172(1995)1080.

227. Ibid.

228. M. Stewart. "Patient Characteristics Which Are Related to Doctor-Patient Interaction." *Family Practice.* 1(1983)30.

229. R. L. Street. "Information-Giving in Medical Consultations: The Influence of Patients' Communicative Styles and Personal Characteristics." *Social Science in Medicine.* 32(1991)541.

230. V. J. Hotz, S. W. McElroy, S. Sanders. "The Costs and Consequences of Teenage Childbearing for Mothers." In *Kids Having Kids: The Consequences and*

Costs of Teenage Childbearing in the United States. Report to the Robin Hood Foundation. Lanham, Md.: University Press of America, 1995.

231. S. E. Mayer. *What Money Can't Buy: Family Income and Children's Life* **233** *Chances.* Cambridge: Harvard University Press, 1997.

232. R. Rector. "Poverty in U.S. Is Exaggerated by Census." *Wall Street Journal.* September 25, 1990, p.A18.

233. H. L. Brown, K. Watkins, A. H. Hiett. "The Impact of the Women, Infants and Children Food Supplement Program on Birth Outcome." *American Journal of Obstetrics and Gynecology.* 174(1996)1279.

234. W. N. Spellacy. "Why WIC?" *American Journal of Obstetrics and Gynecology.* 175(1996)1079.

235. Newsbriefs. "Does Welfare Really Beat Work?" *Roundup.* July 1996, p.7.

236. Ibid.

237. Rector. "Poverty in U.S." p.A18.

238. Aved. "Barriers to Prenatal Care." p.493.

239. R. S. Hunter, N. Kilstrom, E. N. Kraybill, F. Loda. "Antecedents of Child Abuse and Neglect in Premature Infants: A Prospective Study in a Newborn Intensive Care Unit." *Pediatrics.* 61(1978)629.

240. Ibid.

241. Roth. "Crime and Child-Rearing." p.40. Given the significant number of teenage girls who are impregnated by adult males, statutory rape laws should be toughened and enforced. California has already adopted a get tough policy against statutory rape and is currently conducting a public awareness campaign regarding the matter. At the same time, truancy laws and curfews for minors should be more aggressively enforced.

242. Curlender v. Bio-Science Laboratories. 106 California App 3d 811, California Reporter 477, 1980.

243. Stallman v. Youngquist. 152 Illinois App 3rd 683, 504 NE2d 920, 1987.

244. Grodin v. Grodin. 102 Michigan App 396, 301NW2d 869, 1980.

245. L. D. Fleisher. "Wrongful Births: When Is There Liability for Prenatal Injury?" *American Journal of Diseases of Children.* 141(December 1987)1260.

246. J. Trussell, J. A. Leveque, J. D. Koenig, R. London. S. Borden, J. Henneberry, et al. "The Economic Value of Contraception: A Comparison of 15 Methods." *American Journal of Public Health.* 85(1995)494.

247. S. Harlap, K. Kost, J. D. Forrest. *Preventing Pregnancy, Protecting Health: A New Look at Birth Control Choices in the United States.* New York: Alan Guttmacher Institute, 1991.

248. P. R. Lee, F. H. Stewart. "Editorial: Failing to Prevent Unintended Pregnancy Is Costly." *American Journal of Public Health.* 85(1995)479.

249. P. Meskil. "Minorities Fear Contraception." *Medical Herald.* 5, Number 3(April 1995)1.

250. Ibid.

251. Ibid.

252. E. F. Jones, J. D. Forrest, N. Goldman, et al. *Teenage Pregnancy in Indus-*

234   *trialized Countries.* New Haven: Yale University Press, 1986.

253. E. F. Jones, J. D. Forrest, S. K. Henshaw, J. Silverman, A. Torres. *Pregnancy, Contraception and Family Planning Services in Industrialized Countries.* New Haven: Yale University Press, 1989.

254. Meskil. "Minorities Fear Contraception." p.1.

255. P. Meskil. "Unwanted Pregnancies Cost U.S. Millions." *Medical Herald.* 5, Number 4(1995)1.

256. Ibid.

257. Trussell. "The Economic Value of Contraception." p.494.

258. Meskil. "Unwanted Pregnancies Cost U.S." p.1.

259. D. A. Grimes. "A Guest Editorial: Over-the-Counter Oral Contraceptives: An Idea Whose Time Has Not Quite Come!" *Obstetrical and Gynecological Survey.* 50(1995)411.

260. Ibid.

261. Ibid.

262. Anonymous. "OCs o-t-c?" *Lancet.* 342(1993)565.

263. Ibid.

264. Gallup Organization. "Women's Attitudes towards Oral Contraceptives and Other Forms of Birth Control." *Gallup Organization.* January 1994, p.25.

265. Meskil. "Minorities Fear Contraception." p.1.

266. M. A. Lebow. "The Pill and the Press: Reporting Risk." *Obstetrics and Gynecology.* 93(1999)453.

267. E. F. Jones, J. R. Beninger, C. F. Westoff. "Pill and IUD Discontinuation in the United States, 1970–1975: The Influence of the Media." *Family Planning Perspectives.* 12(1980)293.

268. Meskil. "Minorities Fear Contraception." p.1.

269. Ibid.

Index

Abortion, 175–76; ban on, 175; for genetically abnormal fetuses, 17; among minority women, 176; for poor women, 175; services, 175
Abuse, 179
Accidents, 18–20
Acculturation, 166–68; score, 166
Adams, M. M., 164
Adjusted international infant mortality rates, 14
Adolescence, 147–48. *See also* Teenagers
Adolescent pregnancy, 147–49. *See also* Teenage birthrate
Affirmative action, 31
African Americans, 40–41. *See also* Black (race); Black, women
Agency for Healthcare Quality, 142
Ahmed, F., 150
Aid to Families with Dependent Children (AFDC): counterpoint, 69; initial episode of, 154; teen mothers, 150; unwed pregnancy, 155
Air Safety Reporting System, 136
Alabama, 101, 114
Alan Guttmacher Institute, 149, 184
Alcohol, 40–41, 156
Alexander, G. R., 24, 28, 150
Altered expectations, 121–22
Alternative healthcare, 131
American Academy of Family Physicians, 72
American Academy of Pediatrics, 7
American Board of Obstetricians and Gynecologists, 78
American College of Nurse-Midwives (ACNM), 126; Certification Counsel, 126; fostering midwife-based care, 129–31
American College of Obstetricians and Gynecologists (ACOG): cesarean deliveries, 132; domestic violence screening, 75; home uterine activity monitoring, 46; national survey, 85; number of prenatal visits, 7; prematurity prevention, 24; primary care, 72, 73–74; terbutaline pump, 45; bulletins, 54
American College of Physicians, 53

American College of Rheumatology, 97–98
American Institute of Ultrasound in Medicine (AIUM), 48–49
American Medical Association (AMA): prepaid health plans, 103; Sherman Antitrust Act, 102; Socioeconomic Monitoring System, 83
Amini, S. B., 26, 163
Anemia, 66
Annual Survey of Vital Statistics, 15
Antisocial behavior, 150
Arizona, 21, 114–15, 145, 161
Arizona Department of Health Services, 67, 151–52
As Good As It Gets, 109
Association of American Medical Colleges, 72
Attitudes of women, 174
Attorneys, 91. *See also* Lawyers
Australia, 13
Austria, 13
Autopsy studies, 136
Aved, B. M., 85–86, 179

Bailey, J. G., 45
Baker, J., 64
Bakketeig, L. S., 44, 60
Ballantyne, J. W., 33
Baltimore County, Maryland, 63–64
Barber, H. R. K., 91, 109
Baruch, S., 101
Baylor University Hospital, 102
Becerra, J. E., 165
Beckman, H. B., 99
Belgium, 13, 125
Bendectin, 96–97
Benefits package, 105
Bennett, E., 149
Benson, M. D., 149
Berenson, A. B., 146, 156
Binstock, M. A., 7
Biologic plausibility, 40
Birth control pills, 186. *See also* Oral contraception
Birth defects, 15. *See also* Congenital anomalies

241

About the Author

Thomas H. Strong, Jr., was born in 1957 in Baltimore, Maryland, and raised in Butte, Montana. He attended the University of Utah, where he received a B.A. degree in Psychology in 1979 and his medical degree in 1983. Dr. Strong completed his residency in Obstetrics and Gynecology at the University of California at San Francisco's Valley Medical Center in Fresno in 1987. In 1989 he completed a fellowship in Maternal-Fetal Medicine at Los Angeles County/University of Southern California Women's Hospital in Los Angeles. He is board certified in Obstetrics and Gynecology as well as Maternal-Fetal Medicine.

Dr. Strong lives with his wife, Cstephani, in Phoenix, Arizona, where he is Associate Director of Phoenix Perinatal Associates, the largest private Maternal-Fetal Medicine practice in the nation. He has one daughter, Rebekah. Dr. Strong has published or presented more than sixty medical papers in his career and is co-editor of a best-selling medical textbook concerning intensive medical care of pregnant women. He is an Associate Clinical Professor of Obstetrics and Gynecology at the University of Arizona and Assistant Clinical Professor of Obstetrics and Gynecology at the University of California at San Francisco. He is an award-winning speaker and researcher, and has been recognized as an outstanding physician locally (Phoenix Top Docs Award) as well as nationally (Best Doctors in America Award).